W9-BVY-904

Brain Injury
and the

Family

A Life and Living Perspective

Second Edition

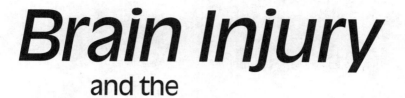

Brain Injury
and the
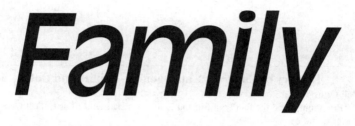
Family

A Life and
Living Perspective

Second Edition

Arthur E. Dell Orto
Paul W. Power

CRC Press
Boca Raton London New York Washington, D.C.

Bayshore

Library of Congress Cataloging-in-Publication Data

Dell Orto, Arthur E., 1943–
  Brain injury and the family: a life and living perspective / Arthur E. Dell Orto, Paul W.
Power.—2nd ed.
    p. cm.
  Prev. ed. published with title: Head injury and the family.
  Includes bibliographical references and index.
  ISBN 0-8493-1325-2 (alk. paper)
    1. Brain damage—Patients—Family relationships. 2. Brain
damage—Patients—Rehabilitation. I. Dell Orto, Arthur E., 1943– Head injury and the
family. II. Power, Paul W. III. Title.
  RC387.5 .D45 2000
  617.4′81044—dc21   99-089634
                                                                                CIP

No claim to original U.S. Government works
International Standard Book Number 0-8493-1325-2
Library of Congress Card Number 99-089634
Printed in the United States of America 1 2 3 4 5 6 7 8 9 0
Printed on acid-free paper

02/05/01

Preface

Brain injury is a serious health care concern because it can happen to anyone we know, love, or care about. It has happened, is happening, and will continue to be part of risk factors associated with the life and living experience. A common ground we all share as human beings is that no one is immune from brain injury — consequently, we are all potential members of the Brain Injury Association. Bergman (1999) places this in a unique context when he states: "If you consider that every person sustaining a brain injury has a circle of support then the reality becomes that brain injury truly touches nearly one out of every ten people in the United States." (p. 1)

With advanced medical technology, an increasing number of persons are surviving and will survive the traumas, but at great physical, emotional, financial, and familial cost. It is estimated that more than 5 million people are living with the effects of traumatic brain injuries; of the 1 million treated in hospitals each year, 230,000 are hospitalized, 80,000 will experience disabilities related to their brain injuries, and 50,000 will die. In addition to the human cost of pain and suffering for people, there are estimated hospital and fatal injury costs of $48 billion annually (Brain Injury Association, 1999; Elovic and Antoinette, 1996). While some costs can be approximated, there is no way of calculating the true costs and enormity of a brain injury.

Since brain injury occurs within a family context, careful consideration must be given to the short-term as well as the long-term impact upon individual family members and the total family unit. When brain injury occurs, the person's family as well as significant others are dramatically affected. Complex and enduring problems of life and living are posed for family members, such as coping with unpredictable behaviors, living with an uncertain treatment outcome, and adjusting to losses associated with this traumatic life experience. Consequently, coping with a brain injury is complex, impacts many domains, and requires meaningful and timely information (Stoler and Hill, 1998). Unfortunately, some families are so overwhelmed by the chaos of brain injury that even though informational resources exist, they may not be perceived as relevant, accessible, or worthwhile.

Even though the family is destabilized and struggling to maintain equilibrium, with meaningful and timely interventions and support, it can still become a vital force in the prevention, treatment, recovery, and rehabilitation process. This is more likely to occur if family needs, assets, potential, and liabilities are understood, appreciated, and attended to from a realistic life and living perspective based upon a vision of hope for all involved.

Because the family and significant others have important roles in both the treatment and rehabilitation process, greater attention must be given to its current state, intergenerational life experiences, quality of life, and future needs. This is most critical because family members are often the victims of the collateral damage related to the trauma of a brain injury.

It is important to realize that brain injury, like other disabilities, casts a very long shadow that can impact, alter, and transform the developmental process of the family, for generations to come (Rolland, 1994).

Brain Injury and the Family: A Life and Living Perspective, Second Edition focuses both on how the family can comprehend, negotiate, adjust, accept, and survive the multidimensional trauma related to a brain injury and become an active partner in the treatment and adaptation process. The content and focus of the material is presented as a partnership with our colleagues, clients, and friends who are living the brain injury experience. A theme of consumer and family relevance connects the chapters which focus on the following topics:

1. Perspective on brain injury
2. Impact of brain injury on the child
3. Impact of brain injury on the adult
4. Impact of brain trauma on the family
5. Assessment
6. Interventions
7. Group counseling
8. Career, work, and employment issues
9. Loss and grief
10. Alcohol and disability
11. Caregiving and respite care
12. Future: hope, needs, and reality

This book is a combination of original material and personal statements by persons and family members living the brain injury experience. This material is supplemented by structured experiential exercises which include discussion questions related to the themes in the book. The original material is presented as a reflection of thoughts based on our professional and personal experiences, prior publications (Dell Orto and Power, 1994; Power 1995; Power and Dell Orto, 1980; Power, Dell Orto, and Gibbons, 1988), and interpretation of the works of others. The personal statements put into perspective issues relevant to treatment, family adaptation, quality of life, and family survival. These statements represent special contributions by our colleagues and friends and create a personalized framework for the material in this book.

The Structured Experiential Tasks (SET) are designed to facilitate the reader's exploration of issues related to the impact of brain injury on the family. These experiences have been systematically developed by the authors with a focus on the major themes from each chapter. An important feature of this book is the appendices which include selected resources related to the needs of survivors, families, significant others, and professionals.

This book is directed toward a family-oriented, life and living perspective. We believe that this perspective is essential in order to create a viable treatment and rehabilitation process that supports and enhances families living with the complexities related to brain injury. We are also aware that for families, brain injury is often in addition to other stressors, problems, and illness in their life. Consequently, some families or individual family members may not be willing, able, or capable to engage in a demanding, rigorous treatment and rehabilitation process, the outcome of which is often unknown. It is from this perspective that the reader will discover ways to involve the family in treatment and also gain perspective into the following questions:

- How does the family influence, impede, or facilitate, the adjustment of a family member who is living with a brain injury?
- What are the limitations and potential limitations of the family?
- What are the resources and potential resources of the family during the treatment and rehabilitation process?
- How can health and human care providers assist the families to maintain balance in their lives as well as attain and maintain a reasonable quality of life?
- How can the recovery and survival of the family as well as the member with a brain injury be facilitated?

While this second edition has been expanded in scope and content, the goal remains similar to our first edition: to better understand the enormity related to coping with brain injury within a familial and life and living context. (Also, to reflect the changes in terminology since the 1994 edition, "head injury" has been changed to "brain injury.") In this edition, the terms "health care professional" and "helper" are used interchangeably to identify those people who, in some way, include in their job or life responsibilities an involvement with the family. Physicians, nurses, personal assistants, social workers, rehabilitation counselors, psychologists, family advocates, physical therapists, occupational therapists, clergy, peer counselors, speech pathologists, and recreational therapists are just some of the groups for whom this book is intended. In the estimation of the authors, all of these people have a unique opportunity to understand and appreciate family dynamics as they affect the person with a brain injury, to provide support for the family, and to share information about effective coping strategies and community resources. The book also originates from and is driven by a rehabilitation and recovery perspective which is essential for a meaningful understanding of what is important to the survivors of brain injuries and their families.

We contend that this is best accomplished while being sensitive to the emerging, changing needs of families challenged by an experience and process that if unchecked can deplete, consume, compromise, and destroy most family systems. This does not imply that the family is flawed because it cannot cope. It does mean that under extraordinary circumstances such as a brain injury, the family needs relevant, and long-lasting support, understanding, and encouragement.

While many accomplishments have been made in brain injury treatment and rehabilitation, much more needs to be done. The challenge is to shape the future, learn from the past, and move from the comfort of what has been accomplished while embracing the imposing reality of what needs to be done.

To place this in context, our frame of reference on where the field is today goes back 20 years to Boston, one of the great medical and rehabilitation centers of the world. For a young woman with a severe brain injury, there were inadequate programs to meet her basic needs. When referrals were made to several prominent rehabilitation programs, the mother of this young person visited the facilities and stated that they were not adequate and, in fact, did not understand the needs of her daughter or any family with a brain-injured member. This mother, driven by her love for her child and frustration with what existed, told us that she would change the system. Frankly, we and other professionals working with her did not have high hopes for change — a response we attribute to limitations in our professional education, which had been more focused on "what was" rather than "what could" or "should be."

In fact, as a result of her vision, change did occur and family needs began to emerge as a factor and force in treatment and rehabilitation. In 1980, Marilyn Price-Spivack co-founded the National Head Injury Foundation and in the process created a new system to meet the needs of those people and families living with a brain injury. It took a concerned, caring, energetic, dedicated mother to begin to challenge and change the system.

However, in the year 2000, as we move into the millenium, we will also bring along some "old problems." Today, and for the foreseeable future, there are and will be those with brain injuries and their families cast adrift in a sea of confusing uncertainty and hope often fueled by desperation. While many problems related to living with and in spite of a brain injury have been solved in the year 2000, others have been created and some are yet to emerge. The bottom line is that some families will be by-passed and ignored. They, in turn, will have to advocate for those in their care, know and expect what they need, and reject that which is inadequate, irrelevant, or unacceptable.

A similar point is made by Berube (1998):

> Traumatic brain injury (TBI) is the leading cause of death and disability among young Americans. It is a phenomenon that requires national attention and vigorous commitment to prevent, treat, and increase understanding. As such, there is great need for advocacy

— for the person with brain injury, caregivers, family members, and rehabilitation professionals — as well as for more education for teachers, employers, politicians, and the public at large. Because each brain injury is as unique as the individual injured, advocates are presented with a formidable task (p. 99).

The actualization of this book is a result of the combined experiences and efforts of many. It is dedicated to Michael Bales and Laura Wilson; Valerie and David Collins, Paul Murphy, who did the impossible by surviving two wars: Vietnam and a brain injury; and Chris Moy, who would not give up hope, and his family, who was there for him. These are people and families who live the experience, are role models, and provide us with invaluable consultation and perspective. We also wish to thank the many persons who provided us with their personal stories of living with the brain injury experience. These personal accounts have brought reality to the theoretical material presented in this book.

We thank Marilyn Price-Spivack, who gave us an idea and a challenge in 1979; Janet Williams for her encouragement; Cheryl Gagne, who added a unique perspective; and Brian McMahon, who pointed the way.

We would also like to acknowledge the technical support of Kevin Berner, Ken Paruti, and Barbara Power, whose skills put the manuscript in order; Barbara Norwitz and Michele Berman of CRC Press, who kept us on task; and our families, who were most understanding during the process.

Arthur E. Dell Orto
Paul W. Power
Boston

References

Berube, J.E. (1998) Brain injury advocacy, *Journal of Head Trauma Rehabilitation*, 13(5), 99–102.

Bergman, A.I. (1999) CDC Report shows prevalence of brain injury, Brain Injury Association's TBI Challenge, June/July, 3(3), 1.

Dell Orto, A.E. and Power, P.W. (1994) *Head Injury and the Family; A Life and Living Perspective*, PMD Publishers Group, Inc., Winter Park, FL.

Elovic, E. and Antoinette, T. (1996) Epidemiology and primary prevention of traumatic brain injury, In: Horn, L.J., Zasler, N.D., editors, *Medical Rehabilitation of Traumatic Brain Injury*, Hanley & Belfus, Philadelphia, pp. 1–28.

Interagency Brain Injury Task Force Report, (1989) National Institute of Neurological Disorders and Stroke, National Institutes of Health, Bethesda, MD.

Marino, M.J. (1999) CDC Report shows prevalence of brain injury, TBI Challenge, Brain Injury Association, 3(3), 1.

Power, P.W. (1995) Family, in *The Encyclopedia of Disability and Rehabilitation*, Dell Orto, A.E. and Marinelli, R.P., Simon & Schuster/Macmillan, New York.

Power, P.W., Dell Orto, A.E., and Gibbons, M. (1988) *Family Interventions Throughout Chronic Illness and Disability*, Springer, New York.

Power, P.W. and Dell Orto, A.E. (1980) *Role of the Family in the Rehabilitation of the Physically Disabled*, Pro-Ed, Austin, TX.

Rolland, J.S. (1994) *Families, Illness and Disability: An Integrated Treatment Model*, Basic Books, New York.

Stoler, D.R. and Hill, B.A. (1998) *Coping with Mild Traumatic Brain Injury*, Avery Publishing, Garden City, NY.

Biography

Arthur E. Dell Orto, Ph.D., C.R.C., is Professor and Chairperson of the Department of Rehabilitation Counseling and Associate Executive Director of the Center for Psychiatric Rehabilitation at Boston University's Sargent College of Health and Rehabilitation Sciences.

He was awarded a B.A. in psychology in 1966 and an M.A. in rehabilitation counseling in 1968 from Seton Hall University. He received a Ph.D. in counseling and rehabilitation from Michigan State University in 1970. Dr. Dell Orto is a licensed psychologist and a certified rehabilitation counselor, whose academic and clinical interests relate to the role of the family in the treatment and rehabilitation process. Dr. Dell Orto teaches a course on The Family and Disability and has given many presentations and workshops focusing on the needs of families living with illness and disability. He is co-editor and co-author with Robert Marinelli of the following books: *The Encyclopedia of Disability and Rehabilitation* (Simon & Schuster, Macmillan Library Reference, 1995), which was awarded an "Excellence in Media Award" by The National Rehabilitation Association; *The Psychological and Social Impact of Disability* (Springer, 1999 and 1991); and *The Psychological and Social Impact of Physical Disability* (Springer, 1984 and 1977). He has co-authored and co-edited with Paul Power: *Head Injury and the Family: A Life and Living Approach* (St. Lucie Press, 1994), which was awarded Pyramid of Distinction and an Award of Excellence by the New England Association of the American Medical Writers; *Illness and Disability: Family Interventions Throughout Chronic Illness and Disability* (Springer, 1988); and *Role of the Family in the Rehabilitation of the Physically Disabled* (Pro-Ed, 1980). He's co-authored and co-edited with Robert Lasky: *Group Counseling and Physical Disability* (Brooks Cole/Duxbury Press, 1979).

Paul W. Power, Sc.D., C.R.C., is Professor and Chairperson of the Counseling and Personnel Services Department, University of Maryland, College Park.

Dr. Power received his M.S. degree in rehabilitation counseling from San Diego State University in 1972 and his Doctor of Science degree from Boston University in 1975. His professional interests have included the role of the family in rehabilitation. He has given national and international workshops on this topic, and has authored or co-authored several books, chapters, and articles on the family and assorted issues in health care. Specifically, he has co-authored and co-edited with Arthur Dell Orto: *Head Injury and the Family: A Life and Living Approach* (PMD Publishers Group, Inc., 1994), *The Role of the Family in the Rehabilitation of the Physically Disabled* (Pro-Ed, 1980), and *Family Interventions Throughout Chronic Illness and Disability* (Springer, 1988). Dr. Power's writings have embraced the topics of career and rehabilitation assessment, mental health counseling, and career planning. With David Hershenson, he co-authored *Community Counseling, Contemporary Theory and Practice.*

Contents

Part II: Interventions

part one

Person and family

chapter one

A perspective on brain injury

The Titanic revisited

Most words and feelings are not adequate enough to capture and express the comprehensive sorrow, pain, anger, concern, desperation, joy, faith, disappointment, rage, love, optimism, and hope shared by persons and families changed and challenged by the impact of a brain injury.

In order to better understand and cope with the complexity related to a brain injury, we must think of it as a condition of living which will give families and society a chance to validate humanity by practicing what we say, demonstrating what we believe, and putting into practice religious principles which help people, gracefully and with dignity, to make the transition from health to illness, illness to disability, loss to gain, and desperation to hope.

Just as the Titanic was considered to be unsinkable and invulnerable by both those who constructed it and those who sailed on her, many families believe that their "family ship" can weather any storm. The problem is that brain injury — and other life challenges — represent more than a storm and includes those unpredictable "icebergs" that can impact families at any time at the most unexpected moment, and often have irreversible consequences. These consequences are often a result of decisions made in times of crisis, based on desperation, and driven by fear and uncertainty.

While the reaction of the family varies according to the severity of the brain injury, subsequent losses, implications and potential for rehabilitation, as well as other factors, a common denominator for families is that they have been changed forever — not necessarily for better or worse, but changed for sure. This change is a result of the initial trauma, the historical and life experiences of the family and the reality of complex and long-term demands placed on or anticipated by the family. In effect, the family has moved to an ecosystem for which they are not prepared and in which the demands are often in excess of the families' resources, supports, and skills. These extreme conditions and unrealistic expectations can rapidly deplete the most resourceful families and magnify their difficulties, which may result in inter-generational, interpersonal, emotional, physical, and financial bankruptcy. This point is reinforced by LaPlante et al. (1996) in their report on the family and disability: "Disability may cause economic hardship that strains families and leads to disruption. It is sometimes said that families in which a member develops a disability experience greater marital dissolution."

The evolving challenge for health and human care personnel, and sys-tems, is to become more aware of and responsive to the needs of families transformed by a brain injury as well as the many other complexities related to the life and living experience (Kosciulik and Pichette, 1996; Perlesz, Kin-sella, and Crowe, 1999; Serio et al., 1997; and Williams and Kay, 1991).

This is critical since most health care and rehabilitation systems are not on the same wavelength as the family and are not primarily designed to meet the changing and emerging needs of families. Connell and Connell (1995) reinforce this point when they state: "Obstacles to coping and recovery exist if medical personnel perceive the illness differently from the patient or the family" (p. 30). This lack of common ground often adds to the stress, strain, and distress experienced by the family forced to let go of a family member and renegotiate a relationship with that individual who is not exactly the person they knew, loved, did not love, and/or cared for prior to injury. Discussing adjustment to health loss, Zemzars (1984) said, "a person can never fully return to his or her pre-illness state of health" (p. 44). This does not mean that gains cannot be made or new goals attained or approx-imated. It does mean — or at least imply — that in many situations all of the consequences related to the loss cannot be fully regained even if this is the driving force of the family or the health care team. A delicate situation occurs if the family has misperceptions regarding potential outcome, espe-cially if they diverge greatly from those of the health care team (Springer et al., 1997).

While we believe in miracles fueled by hope and validated by reality, we also believe that in treatment and rehabilitation families must learn which bridges to cross, which to burn, which to modify, and which to build. Rocchio (1998a) poignantly states: "Let's get one thing straight, there is no cure for brain injury. There is no point at which one is pronounced 'well.' ... It lasts a lifetime. However the good news is that there is life after brain injury and although it may be a difficult life, life after brain injury is worth living" (p. 15).

A familial transformation, consequent to brain injury and other trau-matic events, often occurs during the initial nightmare of emergency room and medical procedures when families or significant others are frequently abandoned, left to fend for themselves, and forced to rely on their meager and faltering resources. The result is that families are terrorized and put at emotional risk in most health care environments that are far from hospitable. This emotional desolation is often the starting point from which families are launched into a potentially unending nightmare that may cover weeks, months, years, or a lifetime.

Anyone who has borne witness to the transformation of a life or the reality of the loss of a loved one in a trauma center or hospital can attest to the aloneness and complexity (Cowley et al., 1994) that are often characteristics of these environments. Support, caring, relevant interventions, and understanding at this point in time are critical.

The starting point or continuation of the long journey of brain injury may be characterized by a loss, potential gain, or increased vulnerability — each of which is influenced by the ability to think clearly and live in a manner that maximizes potential for gain and contains the impact of normative and nonnormative losses and change.

While the sudden and unexpected onset of a traumatic brain injury cannot be undone, nor can the irrational causes, such as violence, be adequately put into perspective (Harrison-Felix et al., 1998), the support needed by families to cope with a brain injury certainly can and must be improved. This is not an easy task in a changing and often hostile health care environment in which corporate profit and greed have taken priority over family survival and patient needs. Rocchio (1998b) addresses this point when she states:

> Because of managed care constraints, family services
> that were once a reimbursable expense now have been
> virtually eliminated. As a result, rehabilitation profes-
> sionals face a daunting challenge in training families to
> manage this responsibility themselves. Insurance carri-
> ers are often more eager to bill services under psychiat-
> ric benefits, which traditionally have low capitation,
> than to provide extended neurorehabilitation which will
> assist family members and individuals with brain injury
> to attain better outcomes and quality of life" (pp. 34–35).

We do not believe that health care and rehabilitation systems are uncaring solely by intent. We do believe that due to the enormity of a brain injury, the complexity of the related problems, and the opportunity, expectation, and pressure for profit, often at any cost, these systems may be forced, by default, into compromised roles. Frequently, families are caught between managed care and managed cost, resulting in "mangled care," which may solve some problems as well as create others. The complexity of these issues is also presented by Rosenthal (1996) in a discussion of rehabilitation ethics, efficacy, myths, measurement, and meaning.

The concerns related to managed care, patient care, quality of care, and related ethical dilemmas are also important issues for the physiatrists working with the brain-injured patients. They are in a very unique position to observe, evaluate, and be impacted by the complexity of the issues and resulting ethical dilemmas (Bontke, 1997).

A flawed, and often convenient, presumption made by some insurance companies, managed care, health care, and rehabilitation systems, is that somehow, and at some time, the family is going to be willing and able to bind its resources and respond to role changes and demanding expectations in order to facilitate the health care, emotional care, treatment, and rehabilitation of a family member or loved one. It is often easier to abrogate responsibility and expect others to fill the voids in an inadequate system.

Unfortunately, not all family members who are brain injured, ill, or well, are "loved ones." The victim may be a family member whose life has been characterized by chaos and dysfunction, whose lifelong behavior prior to the brain injury may have had a central role in causing the family distress. In some cases this was a factor in the cause of the brain injury as well as other losses and traumas. It is important to consider this perspective when attempting to access and involve the family as a resource during the treatment and rehabilitation process when they see it as more of a burden than an opportunity.

This point was illustrated by the following statements by persons faced with the brain injury of a family member:

- What a living hell! My son is one case where we would have been better off if the doctor let him die on the highway. They actually put his brain back in his head and now I must live with a partial person who is killing me emotionally, just as he did before the accident. We would both be better off dead!
- This is not my wife! I did not plan on living my life with someone I do not know or care about anymore. Before this, I was thinking about a divorce — now, I am planning one!
- It is your fault. You bought the motorcycle even though we knew he had a drinking problem. I'll never forgive you!

As intense and as real as these statements are, they can be balanced by the reflections of other families who were able to make more optimistic statements, but still may be in need of support, encouragement, and understanding:

- I will do anything to help my son. Any problem can be solved, any burden can be managed; it is just a matter of perspective. As an engineer I consider problems in need of being solved. Brain injury certainly is a challenging problem!
- My wife is very important to me. Even though she is no longer exactly the same person I married, she was once a great wife and mother and I will never forget that or ever neglect her. I know she would have done the same for me.
- We decided to do the best we can and rely on our friends, family, and faith and practice what we believe in. In some ways our family is closer and stronger after the brain injury — as strange as that sounds.

> It took a major trauma to get all of our attention, and now we focus on what really matters to us — our future together, joy to be had, and peace to be realized.

While these statements differ in emotional content and frame of reference, it is important to realize that, in some cases, open expressions of intense emotion and pain may be more realistic than statements that mask or deny intense feelings. Both are valid frames of reference that indicate where the family has been, where the person is, and where they may have to go.

Feelings related to frames of reference also capture and indicate the significance of familial history, the impact and residuals of familial interaction, and the role of values and traditions on a families' willingness to engage in a demanding and often uncertain outcome of the treatment and rehabilitation process.

Often the present is best understood in the context of the past and its influence on current and future functioning and expectations. Rolland (1994), in discussing a family's illness and disability, emphasizes the importance of understanding the impact of history on current family functioning. He writes, "Organizing a multigenerational assessment within this framework facilitates understanding of the historical interplay of family dynamics and the demands of an illness" (p. 84).

For the family of a person living with a brain injury, the treatment and rehabilitation process is a semi-rational sequence of demands, challenges, disappointments, and rewards. An important question to consider is: where, when, and how are families going to get the support, resources, knowledge, encouragement, role models, and skills they need to negotiate the emotional and physical perils of a changing health care and demanding rehabilitation process?

Recently there has been an increase in the realization that the family is and can become a vital force in negotiating and surviving the brain injury experience. Fortunately, there also has been an increase in information, perspectives, and resources that may make living with, beyond, and in spite of a brain injury more reasonable, bearable, and survivable (Abrahamson and Abrahamson,1997; Appleton and Baldwin, 1998; Boake, 1999; DeBoskey, 1996; Kosciulik and Prichette, 1996; Rosenthal et al., 1998; Williams and Kay, 1991; Williams and Mathews, 1998; Sachs, 1991; Serio et al., 1997). While there is an explosion of research and resources relative to brain injury (Appendices A and B), some of these benefits and services are not accessible or affordable to many people with brain injuries or at their level of changing needs (Stebbins and Leung, 1998).

However, it is important to note that existing systems, models, and programs cannot meet all the needs of all families, all of the time — and it is unreasonable that they are expected to do so. What is not unreasonable is that families should have options, as well as opportunities, to access those resources which can facilitate the conditions of stabilization, acceptance, growth, and recovery.

In some situations the advantage of a personal trauma is that it can create a vision based on what should and could be based — on hopes and dreams, not just resignation. Rolland (1994) made this point when he commented on his medical training: "I did not really learn to appreciate the many dilemmas and strains for families with serious health problems until my personal life was directly affected. Within one year, my mother had a stroke and my first wife was diagnosed with an incurable form of cancer ... I was wholly unprepared for the strains of coping with my family members' life-threatening illnesses" (p. xii).

One of the major challenges of coping with trauma, loss, or brain injury is that people are unprepared for the potentially overwhelming reality that can impact their families. Rolland (1994) emphasizes this point when he states that any family can be expected to "hit the wall" when faced with the extraordinary demands of a chronic illness or disability.

Consequently, most people are vulnerable because they live their lives based upon untested belief systems, and are shocked when their beliefs are not validated by reality. They believe that: illness and disability can, should, and must be prevented, cured, or at least improved; people who are ill and disabled should be cared for, persons with brain injuries should be given access to quality health care; and families should be provided with support and concern. These are beliefs that make people feel good about their humanity and create a frame of reference within which they can interpret the world around them. A major challenge occurs when our expectations are not met, our needs not fulfilled, and our dreams not realized.

However, a critical incident in life and living occurs when individuals and families are "put to the test" and must make the choice to translate beliefs into action. For example, how many people live their lives:

- Believing that their family loves them so much that they will always take care of them regardless of the problems related to a brain injury, illness, or disability
- Making promises that they will never leave each other no matter what challenges, changes, or traumas exist
- Hoping that because they have been self-sacrificing for their children, their children in turn will be equally devoted to them and their family when the need arises
- Living a healthy life style as a means to eliminating illness and disability for themselves or their family
- Relying on laws to prevent crimes of violence that could result in personal or familial loss
- Believing that medical resources will be accessible and improvement possible if enough funding is available and efforts made

When these beliefs are challenged and tested by the reality of illness, disability, and loss in general, or brain injury in particular, individuals and families are often faced with an opportunity to validate their beliefs or recognize that their beliefs may have been untested myths.

Brain injury, like other traumas, illnesses, and disabilities has the potential to challenge familial belief systems because of its complexity, intensity, irrationality, and long-term nature. These characteristics force families to not only examine their beliefs and value systems, but also to make major structured adjustments to accommodate the emerging needs of the family member who has experienced the brain injury and must live with its life-altering effects.

The success or failure of structural adjustments in the family and its members is often determined by the pre-injury lifestyle of the family. Unfortunately, most families do not prepare themselves for the possibility of any illness or disability — certainly not a traumatic brain injury — challenging or eroding their beliefs, values, and resources. Consequently, families are often forced to be reactive to brain injury because they have not based their life perspective on a realistic frame of reference related to the total life and living experience — anything can happen to anyone, what we expect might happen, what we do not expect will.

For example, some people believe that if you take care of yourself physically — eating the proper foods and exercising — you will live a long, healthy life. The reality is that this *may* happen, but the harsher reality is that no matter what we do in this life, we and our loved ones will become ill, disabled, age, and die. Few of us ever think of this reality beyond the cognitive level. We all know this in varying degrees, but most of us are unable to translate it into a functional belief system that permits us to look at life, illness, and brain injury from an opportunistic perspective. For most people, their lives are spent building financial security. They think that if they save money and develop wealth, they will be able to insulate themselves from the ravages of illness and disability as well as their concomitant financial burdens.

While financial resources can make the occurrence of brain injury more bearable, money alone cannot insulate people from the emotional burdens relative to brain injury or other illnesses, traumas, or losses. An additional dimension to the myth of financial security is that in today's economy, many families are forced to spend their resources on long-term care that creates a intergenerational, emotional, and financial bankruptcy. As one parent stated, "I did not save and sacrifice all of my life so that I could pay for coma management for my child. I want to leave something for my other children and my grandchildren apart from bills and resentment." This statement is poignant because it focuses on the intense emotion of a life being dramatically changed and the rupturing of a dream. In today's society, the astronomical costs related to health care of persons with brain injuries have not only created crises for most families, but an opportunity for the public and private sector to take a leadership role in helping individuals and families living the brain injury experience attain and maintain a reasonable quality of life at a reasonable cost.

The challenge is to help families negotiate the perils of life, living, and loss without losing their perspective, purpose, sense of self, and their soul. No burden is too great that it cannot be carried. The goal is to have a meaningful destination and not be forced by default to make the journey alone.

The following personal statement, *Home Run, Not Strike Out*, by Chris and his mother is a multigenerational perspective on a long challenging journey driven by love, hope, and familial concern and commitment. This personal statement is followed by discussion questions and several Structured Experiential Tasks (SET) which are designed to explore selected dimensions of the brain injury experience within a life and living perspective.

Personal statement

Home run, not strike out
by Chris and his mother

Prior to my injury in July 1991, my family had endured its share of trials and tribulations. I guess you could say we were a typical middle class family. At least we considered ourselves middle class. Actually we were on the low income end of middle class, but we were happy. We never felt deprived of anything; even though we didn't have a lot of money for clothes or extras, we never went without. My two older brothers and I shared many wonderful times with our parents. Everyone was always very close: church every Sunday, dinners together, and always discussions on how things were going. My parents, to my knowledge, never missed a sporting event or school function. Everyone was treated fairly, given the same opportunities, and encouraged to grow and learn by experiencing new things. We were always given the freedom to choose our activities, but we were expected not to quit halfway through. If we started something, we were always expected to give it a fair chance before deciding not to continue with it. I guess that's where I developed much of my determination.

My father and mother shared the responsibilities of keeping the household going. When my father lost his job, he took over all the household chores and my mother continued to work full time. Dad was always the athletic type and he instilled in us the belief that hard work, determination, and self-confidence would not only help us athletically, but later in our lives as we began to go out into the world. Our friends were always welcome in our house. I'll never forget how my Dad would fix lunch for me and my best friend during our senior year every day. There aren't too many guys who would want to go home every day for lunch, but I always felt very comfortable with it.

Mom has always been the matriarch of the family. Being an optimist, she is able to see the good in everything. Although she's a small, petite woman, she has a quiet, gentle strength about her. I never tried to "pull one over" on her, since she always had a way of finding things out. When one of us boys would do something we shouldn't have, mom always found out. This still amazes me.

My oldest brother was always quiet and kind of shy. Acting as a role model for me and my other brother, he worked hard in school and pursued extra-curricular activities. At the time of my injury he was out of school and living on his own. As the middle child, my other brother was more aggressive and outgoing. Striving for independence, he couldn't wait to be out on his own. As the youngest of the three boys, I was always on the go. I was very popular in school and gifted athletically. I had just graduated from high school and had secured a baseball scholarship at a nearby university. It had always been my dream to play professional ball. It seemed I had been preparing my *whole life* to play in the "big show." Little did I know that I was really preparing for the challenge of my life.

After graduating from high school I was carefree and looked forward to a great future. I was planning on attending Walsh University, where I had been awarded a baseball scholarship, and majoring in business. I could not wait to start college, become independent, and meet new people. New challenges and new opportunities occupied my thoughts.

The summer after my graduation was a time I remember vividly. Playing 80-some odd games in 6 weeks and enjoying my new freedom with friends, I thought I had it all. I figured as long as I had baseball, friends, and family, I had everything I would ever need. What I did not figure on was losing baseball, being separated from friends, and becoming almost completely dependent on my family.

On July 29, 1991, a friend and I had gone to the mall to do some school shopping. Afterward we decided to hang out at the local strip and see what was going on. We ran into two of our friends, Valerie and Bobby Joe.

The four of us talked and cruised around enjoying the cool summer night. Around 10:30 p.m. we decided to stop off at Taco Bell and go to the restroom and get some drinks. When we entered the Taco Bell I noticed nothing unusual so we proceeded to order. It was supposed to be a fun night out on the town and it probably would have ended that way had the conclusion of the night not found me lying in a coma, fighting for my life.

As we were leaving the restaurant I still hadn't noticed anything unusual. As I proceeded out the door a couple of steps behind my friends, I was struck in the face by a fist. Swinging around to see who had struck me, I was disoriented. As soon as I swung around, I felt a glass bottle shatter over my right temporal lobe. I immediately fell to the ground were I was kicked and beaten for what felt like an eternity, but was actually only a few minutes. Afterward I slowly tried to regain my consciousness. I was rushed to the hospital where I fell into a coma for a month.

Emerging from my coma was the greatest challenge of my life, a challenge I will never forget. It called for every resource I had if I were to breathe and walk again. It was like I was alone in a dense, thick fog groping for a familiar hand, yet unable to find anything concrete and strangely aware of vast emptiness and solitude. This is a faint reflection of my coma. As I lay there, I experienced repeated flashes of light … my brain inevitably reacted. I wondered where the light came from! Had I really seen it or was it only a figment of my imagination? I convinced myself that the flash of light was real and, thus, my only hope of finding my way back home. From a great distance, I heard the distinct voices of my mother, father, brothers, and the girl next door, Amy. Each time I heard their encouragement, I drew one step closer to the light. Although I felt like falling into despair, a word of love from God, my family, and my friends urged me forward. Without such love I would not have advanced even one step. Along with these words of love, I also heard the muffled voices of doctors and the high-pitched whispers of nurses as they wondered what they could do to help me. Eventually, they concluded that I would not make it. I was determined to prove them wrong.

Every day, I fought the coma with all of my might. Every day, I drew a little closer to the light. Finally, the day came when I opened my eyes and saw the heartbroken tears of the people I loved and longed to be with. Meanwhile, I could not move a single muscle in my body. I could not even talk. However, this did not bring my spirits down; somewhere deep within I knew that I had just answered the greatest challenge of all, the challenge of coming back from virtual death.

After awakening from my coma I slowly began to realize what had happened. I went from a fully functional young adult to practically a vegetable in a blink of an eye. I was left totally immobile, not able to talk and my world had seemed to crumble to dust. My family and friends were there to support me; if not for them I think I would have died.

During the ensuing weeks, the doctors and nurses gave me little hope for recovery, but through persistent pleading, my mother convinced the doctors to give me time before decisions were made to institutionalize me. My family and I vowed to meet this brain injury head on and give it our best. I slowly regained mobilization and could see gradual improvements. The doctors also saw my progress and decided to send me to a rehabilitation hospital to continue therapy.

It was at the rehabilitation hospital that my attitude and commitment to recovery preceeded all other thoughts. My family, friends, therapist, nurses, and doctors were my team and they were counting on me to bring them to victory. You see, it was the ninth inning, the game was tied, the bases were loaded, and I was at the plate facing a full count. It was the kind of situation I thrived on. It was do or die time. I could dig in, face the challenge, and try, or I could drop my bat, strike out, and die. The choice was mine. What did I do? Well, I stepped in the box, dug my feet in good, and my mind focused on the pitcher, or in this case the injury. I saw the ball coming; it was like a balloon. I stepped into the ball, made a smooth swing, and then I heard a crack. The ball ricocheted off my bat like a bullet from a gun. I just stood there and watched it soar high and long; I knew in an instant it was gone. As I touched each base, a part of my recovery passed, and before I knew it, I was home, starting school, and enjoying life again.

Although my recovery is not yet complete, I play a game every day in my head, and with every hit, catch, and stolen base, a part of my recovery passes. My next home run could be the one that brings me full circle. The pursuit of this dream is encompassed by the determination and hope that one day I will make it back to my ballfield. All I can do is try and pray that everything will turn out right, and if it does not, I will still go on because I know I gave it my best.

The road to recovery has been long and wearisome, but I have already put many miles behind me and I know I will emerge completely triumphant. This experience has taught me many valuable lessons. Above all, it has convinced me that the human will can overcome obstacles that many consider insurmountable. I have walked through the valley of the shadow of death and have come out, not unscathed but undaunted. I am among the few people who can say that they have experienced near-death and were able to live and talk about it. I consider myself lucky and remain grateful to all who have helped me recover from this disaster. My experience has indisputably helped make me the person I am today.

Although many things helped my family overcome this catastrophe, the most helpful was first and foremost, our faith in God and belief that He would make everything all right. Second was the overwhelming support we received from family and friends. How could we not make it with such kindness and compassion? Third was becoming knowledgeable about brain injury. This seemed to make us feel more in control of the situation, instead of relying on doctors and nurses for details of what was happening. Throughout the injury, we kept a positive outlook on life, knowing that we would pull through. The family, as a whole, had a kind of inner strength, which told each member things would work out in the end. Finally, we came to accept the situation and the consequences it has brought. The past cannot be changed, but the present and future can.

Intervention was never offered to my family. I often wonder why, but I guess no one ever thought to ask what the family needed. Intervention that would have been helpful to my family includes:

- A team of doctors that would offer in-depth knowledge on the subject of head injury, or offer literature or reading material in lay-person's terms
- Counseling for family because just being able to talk to someone about what was happening would have helped. Information on support groups and meeting other families who have experienced such trauma, would have been extremely soothing
- Someone offering assistance with a list of attorneys, if needed, or other medical facilities better equipped and able to help patient progress
- Someone who would have been able to structure a program that would have fit my family's needs, for example, phone numbers of groups or organizations that offer help, and if out of town, assistance with lodging, meals, churches, etc.

After reading and realizing the lack of professional help my family had, I have to wonder what really helped us get through this experience. It seemed everything that was needed by the family, the family provided. I thank God for giving us the strength, courage, and wisdom to endure each day and for watching over us as we struggle through head injury.

Mother's perspective

I remember lying in bed the night we got the phone call. I was wondering why Chris was late. It was 10:30 p.m. He had gone school shopping at the mall with a friend. It wasn't like him not to call if he was going to stop somewhere else.

Just the weekend before, he had finished up a grueling summer baseball schedule, playing 80-some odd games in 6 weeks. He had worked so hard on getting a scholarship and we were very proud of him. I remember his last tournament game. When they lost, he quickly tossed his uniform, like only a ball player could, to get ready for the drive to Walsh University where he would be attending in the Fall. It was orientation weekend, but he had come back to play his final game. His dad had said, "Well, Chris, that was your last game." A strange feeling passed through me, and I quickly added, "Until you get to college." As we later drove to the hospital that night, that conversation kept floating through my thoughts.

We really didn't know how bad things were until we arrived at the hospital. When they told us he was having seizures and would need immediate brain surgery, we were devastated. Some friends of ours had gone through a similar experience just the year before, so were all too aware of the seriousness of the situation. As friends and family gathered at the hospital to keep a constant vigil, the pain and devastation set in. So many questions kept going through our minds. Would he live? If he did, how would he be? Why was this happening to us? The nurses were very helpful and brought much-needed comfort during the long weeks while he was in a coma. My husband and I could not bear to leave the hospital. The doctors did not seem to be educated enough to deal with the situation, so we finally had to make the agonizing decision to have him moved. All along we prayed to God to give us the strength, courage, and wisdom to make the right decisions.

My husband was offered a job, and the decision was made for him to go to work as I stayed with Chris. My husband quickly took over all the responsibilities of working and running the household, plus handling all the stacks of paperwork. I, on the other hand, was learning, right along with Chris, about therapy. Together we struggled to help him get better. For him, it was a matter of working relentlessly to make his body do what he wanted it to do. For me, it was the anguish of watching and being there for my child, but not really being able make it all better. It was a feeling of helplessness. I was determined to learn everything I could about head injury. Somehow being more knowledgeable on the subject made me feel more in control. I always tried to keep a cheerful, encouraging face on for Chris even though my heart was breaking. My other two sons were great. The middle son remained at home with his father and did everything he could to help out. My oldest son visited Chris daily and opened his bachelor apartment, which he was sharing with two other guys, to his mother.

Although the outlook was bleak, we never gave up hope that Chris would return to normal. But as we've learned, nothing is ever normal. Our lives are constantly changing. As Chris begins to have more and more control over his body, he seems more content. When Chris started school again after his injury I never imagined he would do this well or go this far. Having him transfered so far from home has been hard on the whole family, but he seems so happy that it's hard not to be happy for him. From the beginning, he was always accepted for who he was, not for what his body had trapped him into. The son we had was taken from us, but the son we were given back is even better in so many ways. Chris is a constant inspiration to all who come in contact with him. There is not a doubt in my mind that he will succeed in life.

As I reflect back, the pain and hurt will never go away, but I developed a tolerance for it. Life for all of us in this world is a challenge. You draw strength to meet those challenges through those around you. Things are so unpredictable, but would we really want to know how things will turn out? All we can hope for is to be surrounded by love, and the courage to face what life has to offer. A Garth Brooks song better explains this point: "Yes my life is better left to chance. I could have missed the pain, but I'd of had to miss the dance."

Epilogue

Today Chris is working, married, and has a child, and that has made it all worthwhile.

Discussion questions on the personal statement

1. If you were engaged and your fiancée had a traumatic brain injury, what would you do? What would your family suggest?
2. How would you respond if you or a family member was brain injured as a result of violence?
3. Discuss the athletic frame of reference that Chris had and how it was an asset in treatment, recovery, and rehabilitation.
4. Why was Chris' family able to rally in a time of crisis?
5. If your loved one was not expected to survive, what would you do if faced with the decision on life supports?
6. After reading this personal statement, would you consider rehabilitation at any cost?
7. What would your response be if you and your family made every effort possible to "normalize" your brain-injured family member even if he remained at a two-year-old's level of functioning?

8. Define and discuss quality of life. Discuss any future issues that may occur.
9. What did Chris mean when he stated, "I know I gave it my best."
10. How can people learn to adapt to change as Chris and his family did?

Set 1. Curing traumatic brain injury

Perspective

What if an experimental drug were discovered that could eliminate most of the effects of a traumatic brain injury and restore a person to almost pre-injury levels of functioning? The cost is $50,000 per year.

Exploration

1. Who should pay for the drug?
2. How should people be selected for treatment?
3. Should severity of injury be considered?
4. What if a person had a dual disability such as traumatic brain injury and severe mental illness?
5. Should a company be limited in the amount of money it could charge for such a drug?

Set 2. How long? How old?

Perspective

A severe brain trauma may last months or years. This long-term perspective often can influence the process of making decisions and living with the consequences.

Exploration

1. How long should a 10-year-old child be kept in a coma management unit? A 38-year-old person? A 78-year-old person?
2. What factors must be considered in making these decisions?
3. What does "forever" mean to families who are responsible for the emotional and financial well-being of a family member with a brain injury?
4. How long should parents be responsible for a child?
5. How long should children be responsible for parents?
6. Should families be required to pay for medical and rehabilitation services if gains are not made?
7. Should long-term care facilities be required to keep a patient after funds are exhausted?

Set 3. Is the person with a brain injury more important than the family?

Perspective

The occurrence of a severe disability in general and a brain injury in particular often focuses all of the family's emotional resources on the person who has sustained the injury. Often this focusing is essential to contain the fallout from the injury as well as to stabilize the total family system. However, in order for families to realign their goals and to establish a different balance in their lives, they must make a transition that considers the individual needs of family members, the total needs of the family and the emerging, changing needs of the family member challenged by a brain injury.

Exploration

1. In coping with the demands of a brain injury in your family, how did/would you allocate emotional resources?
2. Is it ever possible to regain balance in the family following a brain injury?
3. How long is a long time?
4. If you had a severely disabled child, a parent with Alzheimer's Disease, or a brain-injured spouse, how would you allocate your emotional resources?

References

Abrahamson, P. and Abrahamson, J. (1997) *Brain Injury: A Family Tragedy*, HDI, Houston, TX.

Appleton, R. and Baldwin, T. (1998) *Management of Brain Injured Children*, Oxford University Press, New York.

Berube, J.E. (1998) Brain injury advocacy, *J. of Head Trauma Rehabil.*, 13(5), 99–102.

Boake, C. (1999) Family articles for traumatic brain injury: choosing appropriate placement facilities, *Commun. Skill Build.*, Tucson, AZ.

Bontke, C.F. (1997) Managed care in traumatic brain injury rehabilitation: physiatrist's concerns and ethical dilemmas, *J. of Head Trauma Rehabil.*, 12(1), 37–43.

Connell, G.M. and Connell, L.C. (1995) In hospital consultation: systemic intervention during medical crisis, *Fam. Syst. Med.*, 13(1), 29.

Cowley, R.S., Swanson, B., Chapman, P., Kitik, B.A., and Mackay, L.E. (1994) The role of rehabilitation in the intensive care unit, *J. of Head Trauma Rehabil.*, 9(1), 32–42.

DeBoskey, D.S. (1996) *Coming Home: A Discharge Manual for Families of Persons with a Brain Injury*, HDI Publishers, Houston, TX.

Harrison-Felix, C., Zafonte, R., Mann, N., Dijkers, M., Englander, J., and Kreutzer, J. (1998) Brain injury as a result of violence: preliminary findings from the traumatic brain injury model systems, *Arch. of Phys. Med. and Rehabil.*, 79.

Kosciulik, J.F. and Prichette, E.F. (1996) Adaptation concerns of families of people with head injuries, *J. of Appl. Rehabil. Counseling*, 27(2), 8–13.

LaPlante, M.P., Carlson, D., Kaye, H.S., and Bradsher, J.E. (1996) Families with disabilities in the United States, Disability Statistics Report (8), U.S. Department of Education, National Institute on Disability and Rehabilitation Research, Washington, D.C.

Perlesz, A., Kinsella, G., and Crowe, S. (1999) Impact of traumatic brain injury on the family: a critical review, *Rehabil. Psychol.*, 44(1), 6–35.

Rocchio, C. (1998a) The unvarnished truth, there is no cure for brain injury, *Family News and Views*, Brain Injury Association, 15–16.

Rocchio, C. (1998b) Can families manage behavioral programs in home settings, *Brain Injury Source*, Brain Injury Association, 2(4), 34–35.

Rolland, J.S. (1994) *Families, Illness and Disability*, Basic Books, New York.

Rosenthal, M. (1996) Traumatic brain injury rehabilitation ethics and efficacy: myths, measurement and meaning, *J. of Head Trauma Rehabil.*, 11(1), 88–95.

Rosenthal, M., Griffith, E., Kreutzer, J., and Pentland, B. (1998) *Rehabilitation of the Adult and Child with Traumatic Brain Injury*, 3rd ed., F.A. Davis, Philadelphia.

Sachs, P.R. (1991) *Treating families of brain-injured survivors*, Springer-Verlag, NY.

Serio, C., Kreutzer, J.,Witol, A. (1997) Family needs after traumatic brain injury: a factor analytic study of the family needs questionnaire, *Brain Injury*, 11, 1–9.

Springer, J.A., Farmer, J.E., and Bouman, D.E. (1997) Misperceptions, mishaps and pitfalls in working with families after traumatic brain injury, *J. of Head Trauma Rehabil.*, 12(6), 63–73.

Stebbins, P. and Leung, P. (1998) Changing family needs after brain injury, *J. of Rehabil.*, 64(4), 15–22.

Stoler, D.R. and Hill, B.A. (1998) *Coping with Mild Traumatic Brain Injury*, Avery Publishing, Garden City, NY.

Williams, J.M. and Kay, T. (Eds.) (1991) *Head Injury: A Family Matter*, Paul H. Brooks Publishing Company, Baltimore.

Williams, J.M. and Mathews, M. (1998) Independent Living and Brain Injury, Research and Training Center on Independent Living for Underserved Populations, University of Kansas, Lawrence, KS.

Zemzars, I.S. (1984) Adjustment to health loss: implications for psychosocial treatment, in Community Health Care for Chronic Physical Illness: Issues and Models, Milligan, S.E., Ed., Case Western Reserve University, Cleveland, 44–88.

chapter two

Brain injury and the child/adolescent reaction

The most common cause of acquired disability in childhood and adolescence is traumatic brain injury (TBI) (Kehle and Clark, 1996). It is estimated that 100,000 children 14 years of age and younger are hospitalized each year with serious brain injuries (Kraus, Rock, and Hemyari, 1990). Falls and child abuse account for the majority of younger children who are injured, while automobile accidents cause the majority of adolescent brain injuries (Hux and Hacksley, 1996). Mild brain injuries, which are 95% of the brain injuries sustained annually by approximately 1 million children and adolescents (Hux and Hacksley, 1996), tend to be time limited. Moderate to severe brain injuries, however, result in chronic and late onset symptomalogy affecting long-term lifestyle and developmental milestones (Patrick and Hostler, 1998). Outcomes after brain injury are a complex mix of natural recovery, individual characteristics and adjustment patterns, and unique stressors to parents and other family members. Children and adolescents who experience brain injury traumas have a unique array of behavioral and emotional reactions (Michaud et al., 1993; Guthrie, Mast, and Richards, 1999). With pediatric brain injury, parental hopes for the child's or adolescent's future are commonly destroyed. Extra demands created by the young person's disability may strain marital relationships and engender continued conflict over caregiving issues (Camplair et al., 1990).

A troubling issue to the study of adjustmental patterns to brain injury, however, is that one of the singular features of pediatric brain injury can be the delayed onset of symptoms, appearing months or even years following the trauma (Patrick and Hostler, 1998). Such a delay can change the understanding of what determinants actually influence a specific, behavioral reaction. To achieve some clarity in what is a complex adjustment situation, it is more appropriate to understand child and adolescent brain injury in a psycho-social context, in which the health care provider team, the peer/social group, the school, and the family contribute to the individual's quality of life.

This chapter will identify significant determinants to the child's and adolescent's reactions to a brain injury, including an identification of the influences on the young person's life adjustment. The problems for the young person that emerge from the trauma of brain injury will be discussed. This chapter will also explain the dominant themes in the adolescent and child reaction, identify the unique stressors on the family resulting from the brain injury, and describe selected factors conducive to good adjustment which can assist the younger person to maintain a reasonable quality of life. Determinants, reactive themes, and helping strategies are all interconnected. Effective interventions build upon an understanding of both the causes and reactions.

Determinants and influences on child/adolescent reaction and life adjustment to brain injury

Both determinants and influences to the emotional reaction to a brain injury should be viewed in a developmental perspective. The impact of an injury can be more or less problematic depending on the stage of development and expression of any given skill for the age and individual differences of that person at that particular time. The child's and adolescent's life adjustment patterns need to be interpreted within the context of the developing individual with the assumption that injury to the developing brain may have more severe long-term and delayed onset of effects (Lazar and Menaldino, 1995). Younger children, moreover, may be more vulnerable to severe effects from head traumas than adolescents because they may have less fully developed life skill bases. Because of these developmental differences, understanding the emergence of individual reactions is complex. There is mixed agreement on which determinants can predict behaviors and conduct problems (Patrick and Hostler, 1998). There are certain determinants that represent themes found in pre-injury and injury characteristics of young people which can provide guidelines to understanding brain injury related behaviors.

Severity of injury

Young people with brain injuries show a positive relationship between severity of injury and changes to motor-sensory skills, communications, and intellectual functioning (Patrick and Hostler, 1998). In turn, modifications in motor-sensory skills, communication patterns, and cognitive skills can affect impulse control and the way an individual manages his anger and frustration. These neuro-behavioral changes can facilitate depressive episodes with the accompanying lack of motivation to undertake many life tasks or to engage in necessary social relations. Since decreased motor coordination is commonly associated with a brain injury, this physical aspect of the disability may be particularly important for adolescents who are very concerned with body image.

Age at the time of injury

Overlapping with the neuro-developmental level of the young person is age. Age can determine how the child or adolescent confronts returning to school following a trauma and how he engages in complex and advanced learning challenges. There are certain developmental tasks associated with age groups, and how one has learned these tasks prior to an injury can make a difference in post-injury adjustment. The concept of age includes the emotional adjustment of the young person at the onset of the injury. A secure child who believes he is warmly accepted by his parents may adapt more easily to the limitations imposed by a brain injury than someone who has conflictual feelings or perceives a clear sense of rejection regarding parental acceptance. A child's competence and self-esteem are strongly affected by experiences in the family circle.

In adolescence the move toward independence becomes a powerful driving force. However, an individual who is coping with brain injury effects and who requires assistance with many activities of daily living is likely to feel disempowered, threatened, and vulnerable. Identity issues may also be aggravated as a result of the injury. The concept of identity includes self-confidence, self-esteem, and a sense of how one is perceived by others. At the onset of brain injury, these perceptions may tend to be negative. For an adolescent who is coping with the effects of a brain injury and who may be less self-assured there is additional difficulty in resolving questions emerging from maintaining self-esteem. Combined with these issues of identity are the daily challenges of satisfying the need for companionship and peer support. Because of mental and behavior deficits associated with brain injury, social inclinations become frustrating or unrealistic. The individual may have trouble with the skills required to maintain group relations and may even become a stranger to convivial, good fellowship.

Academic issues

School environment plays a role in the identification with those who have academic skills and goals. A child's self-perception of competence is strongly affected by his experience in the school environment. School factors, consequently, play a key role in the young person's reaction to a brain trauma (Miller, 1995; Clark, Russman, and Orme, 1999). Re-entry into the school system can be a very significant hurdle to overcome (Clark, 1996). The cognitive dysfunction resulting from a TBI can drastically change an individual's learning ability, especially in the academic domains. Problems with academic achievement may not be apparent for a year or more after injury, so when they are detected they may not be attributed to the injury. The young person can experience frustration due to sudden change in academic performance and confusion associated with repeated failure at tasks which were not difficult prior to the injury. Lazar and Menaldino (1995) believe that during the school years difficulties may emerge when the young person confronts transition points, such as when he makes the change from learning to read to reading to learn. These difficulties may cause children and adolescents to re-evaluate their roles and expectations. Clark (1996) believes that most students living with head injuries initially view themselves the way they were, not the way they are when returning to school. When faced with newly acquired deficits, survivors and their families may be forced to change their expectations of themselves.

With the growing number of young people with TBI entering the educational system, challenges emerge regarding the educator's knowledge as to how a brain injury can affect a student's academic and social functioning. It has been reported that a majority of teachers do not want survivors of a brain injury in their classroom (Hux and Hacksley, 1996). Socio-cultural conditioning, unstructured situations, and the societal emphasis on personal productiveness and achievement may contribute to both anxiety and negative attitudes from teachers. Academic deficits displayed by survivors of TBI conflict with achievement values, not only causing discomfort in teachers, but frustration and perhaps a sense of rejection in the young person.

The family environment

The family has a decided influence on the young person's adjustment to a brain injury (Wade, Taylor, and Drotar, 1998). The family's adjustment can be a primary determinant for the emotional adaptation of the youth with mild to moderate brain injury. Pre-injury family functioning is the best predictor of positive family adjustment in both children and adults, even more so than injury severity (Pieper, 1991). Family instability, parent psychiatric history, socio-economic status, child-rearing practices, and parental expectations all contribute to post-injury quality of life. Parents who have available support resources, stability, and education may minimize the at-riskness for dysfunctional adjustment patterns. The parent's emotional resources can be drained by caregiving demands, leaving little time for the adjustment demands of their other children. Parents who have a developed ability for tolerance and empathy and who understand the effects of brain injury and the distinctive needs of their other children contribute to a home environment that is more conducive to the caregiving demands of the child who is brain injured.

Frequently lost in any discussion of family dynamics and brain injury is the reaction of siblings to a TBI. There has been little information reported on sibling adjustment to head injury. Studies have suggested that the greater the impairment and dependence of a family member who is handicapped, the poorer the adjustment of his non-handicapped siblings (Waaland, 1990). Birth order, gender, and family size may also be predictive of objective and subjective burden and socio-emotional adjustment of non-handicapped siblings. Such issues as embarrassment of the behavior of the brother or sister, guilt for not being the injured one, and resentment for not receiving as much attention as the injured, are concerns that impact the family. Further distress occurs when the children become the sounding board for their parent's grief and frustration, especially when there is a single parent (Patterson, 1988). Siblings, consequently, may be at increased risk for a multitude of adjustment problems. These problems cause stress within the family environment which, in turn, affect the adjustment of the young person with head injury. Yet attitudes from parents which emphasize the importance of basic trust and cooperation may decrease sibling problems and help the young person develop effective coping mechanisms.

Severity of the injury, age at time of onset, academic issues, and the family environment can influence how the young person will adapt to the effects of a brain injury. Such factors as pre-injury adjustment, the length of the coma, and threats to the emotional needs of the young person, i.e., love and affection, self-respect, achievement, independence, and acceptance, may also contribute to the manner of the child's or adolescent's life adjustment. The trauma can eventually trigger a wide variety of emotions, all of which must be considered when helping the family to assist a family member to manage the demands of living with the disability.

Dominant reactions and problems which emerge from child/adolescent brain injury

As a result of the brain trauma there are many physiological changes to the individual, such as motor-sensory skills, communication and intellectual functioning, and the emergence of behavioral and psycho-social problems. Many deficits, as stated earlier, may appear at a later point when certain functions and skills do not develop as expected. An understanding of the emotional reaction of the young person must be viewed in the context of these physiological changes, as well as the family "climate" and the attitudes of professionals toward the young person and the family.

When discussing the young person's reaction to a brain trauma, particular attention should be directed to the adolescent. Adolescents have the task of discovering their identity, separating from their parents, and searching for independence. An injured adolescent has the further challenge of integrating the reality of a brain injury and the limitations it imposes on identity development. Young people can become more anxious about their futures, especially concerning social relationships, careers, and adult lifestyles. This anxiety may mesh with a kind of denial of their post-injury conditions (Patterson, 1988). When attempts at independence are thwarted because of the residual effects of a brain injury, the adolescent may become angry and rebellious. Consequently, independence becomes a painful issue for the young person. They struggle with the symptoms of brain injury that are not that visible and with the independence to perform select, adult social roles.

The ultimate deprivation for the child or adolescent may be the loss of a normal life span and fantasies about the way life should be (Patterson, 1988). The impact of this loss may arise during the re-adjustment period to school demands or the frequent interaction with peers. The losses could be both interactive and cumulative. Progressive realization that now life is different and one no longer has the developed ability to capably perform many activities of daily living may lead to greater social isolation and psychological loss as self-esteem and hope diminish (Patterson, 1988).

Though depression is considered a significant consequence for adults after TBI (Rosenthal et al., 1998), it is also found in young people who may be having difficulties resuming a productive life and maintaining satisfactory interpersonal relations. Adolescents may become withdrawn and have intense feelings of disappointment, frustration, and anger; they feel there is little satisfaction that can be derived from life. A shroud of bleakness and self-doubt may also invade the cognitive and emotional life of young people. All in all, the depression may manifest itself as sadness, irritability, or impaired cognition (Barrett, 1999).

This change in conduct is due to their restricted ability to understand many daily adjustment demands, a reduced ability for planning and self-reliance, and a difficulty to remain focused on tasks. Because of these changes young people with brain injuries will show increased irritability, frustration, social isolation, impulsiveness, anxiety, phobias, and frequent anger (Donders and Ballard, 1996). Though sensori-motor disorders in childhood often are transient relative to more persistent cognitive disorders, adolescents, in particular, will experience a sense of powerlessness and may project feelings of hostility. These feelings are often projected onto other family members who are perceived as the angry ones. The individual's anxiety emerges from the daily stresses, conflicts, and difficulties associated with unresolved problems. Fears might arise from school and social problems and the worries caused by a lack of self-confidence. Moreover, the child or adolescent's early experiences in life while coping with a brain injury, will have a profound effect on later functioning. The attitudes of parents and professional workers that a child or adolescent's emotional reaction to a brain trauma is significant and merits consideration is an important variable in the outcome of the young person's adjustment process (Miller, 1995).

Unique stressors on the family resulting from child/adolescent brain trauma

The emotional reactions of the young person with a brain injury can precipitate serious difficulties for family members, health providers, and school personnel. The adolescent's developmental struggles with sexual awareness, independence-dependence conflict, and understanding of his own values and lifestyle as being distinct from his parents, can cause continued family anxiety, disruption of family patterns, and altered parent and sibling roles. Prolonged medical treatment can intensify the individual's conflict of separation, affecting the expectations of parents toward him. The young person's impulsivity, frustration, risk taking, labile moods, memory impairments, poor judgment, difficulties following directions, a tendency to interrupt others in conversation, and social isolation can create tension within the family environment and inhibit the family's attempts to "right itself" and re-establish a working balance among all family members.

Because of the implications for future planning for the young person with a brain trauma, the family realizes that hopes and dreams may have to be changed. Such a transition represents a loss for family members, who grieve over the reality of long-term brain injury symptoms. With grief comes anger, frustration, disappointment, and depression among family members.

The young person's re-entry into the family, school, and neighborhood communities often stimulates another transitional crisis in the family. Though the child's return home and successful re-entry depends upon a close relationship between family dynamics and the child's individual behavioral integrity (Patrick and Hostler, 1998), during this transition marital conflicts, inappropriate family alliances, and unhealthy coping strategies tend to be heightened. Avoiding adjustment demands, denying the reality of the behavioral symptomalogy, and displacing parental frustration on other children can only add to family disruption. Moreover, during the community re-entry phase the family may still be wondering about future prognosis, seeking complete information on the young person's problems, and figuring whether there are adequate resources to manage rehabilitation needs.

All in all, there are cognitive, emotional, and behavioral demands on the marital relationship. This is usually combined with large financial burdens. These demands create a difficult time for families, especially those with young children in a persistent, vegetative state or coma since this can become indefinite. Understanding complex information about a brain injury, being uncertain about the course of the illness, worrying over the future of the now "less than perfect child," and accommodating lives to the caring needs of the child represent stressors that cause a large burden on the marital relationship. Necessary changes to the roles, rules, and routines of family life to accommodate the needs of the young person with a brain injury have an impact on the whole family as a systemic unit (Patterson, 1988; MacFarlene, 1999).

From these stressors emerge selected needs for the family which must be recognized by family members and health professionals if the family is to achieve an appropriate level of adjustment.

Family needs emerging from brain injury

A significant study reported on how over 200 families with children with TBI responded to inquiries about their needs at the present time (Pieper, 1991). The highest ranked needs were:

1. To have my questions answered honestly
2. To have complete information on my child's problems with memory and communication as well as such physical problems as weakness, headaches, dizziness, and visual or walking difficulties

3. To have explanations from professionals given in terms that family members can understand
4. To have enough resources for my child, such as rehabilitation programs and counseling
5. To have a professional to turn to for advice or services when my child needs help
6. To have complete information on the medical care of the child's disorder

Accurate, clear information and support services appear to be central to the needs of these parents. Families also need someone at the very beginning of the brain injury trauma to give them appropriate relevant, helpful medical information, emotional support, and practical guidance. Support services could include information and referrals, supportive counseling, and training in caregiving, stress reduction, and financial management. Special education was marked in the questionnaire as an essential service. Interestingly, when parents were asked about those services which could have been requested if they were known at injury onset, the highest demands were support groups, free health maintenance organizations, financial counseling, sibling counseling, and family counseling.

Many of these needs, of course, often go unmet, and this situation only contributes to family tension as attempts are made to manage daily living demands. When the child or adolescent re-enters the family after a prolonged hospitalization, and family members are confronted with the reality of the disability, expectations must be modified, special education classes should be arranged, case management concerns need attention, and sibling and parental roles are altered. Other needs surface, moreover, for family members during the post-acute rehabilitation phase. They include the assurance that their family member will be safe, allaying fear of the future, issues around adequate rehabilitation or medical insurance coverage, understanding the rehabilitation process, and the realization that they are making a positive contribution to their loved one's care (Coppa et al., 1999).

Disturbances to child behavior, i.e., impulsivity and frustration leading to anger, can be the most challenging of all the brain trauma symptoms (Patrick and Hostler, 1998). In attempting to fulfill their unmet needs, and at the same time manage the everyday demands of living with a child with brain injury, families come to a crossroads. Family life can deteriorate, become more rewarding, or families can deteriorate and then restore themselves to productive, satisfying living. There are a number of factors conducive to a reasonable adjustment for family members. They are:

1. **A stable family situation**
   Though living with a young person with a brain injury can be continually disruptive, open communication among family members, a sense of security among siblings, a trusting, caring relationship among spouses, and a coping ability to at least manage difficult situations

and perhaps capitalize on successes, all contribute to a stable family life. Such stability does not discount unexpected periods of crisis, but a crisis has a greater probability of being managed successfully by a family that is stable, cohesive, and flexible.

2. **Parent-child relationship predominately positive**

   The characteristics of this relationship include a "basic trust" established in the child, and a sensitivity to the young person's needs. With frequent behavior-related episodes, it may be very difficult to nurture this trust, but the nurturing flows from convictions that "we" want what is best for our child. An awareness of the child's or adolescent's current and emerging needs is important in building a working relationship between parent and child.

3. **Parents and professionals working cooperatively, and not at cross-purposes**

   Such a factor presumes good communication between the professional and family members, a communication that includes realistic information available to the young person and family about the nature of the brain injury, accessible medical, educational, and financial resources, and a clear response to questions. Parents report continued difficulties with professionals over communication issues, and health providers need to be aware of parental information needs and the ability of parents to interpret information.

4. **Adequate opportunities for the young person to have peer contact and other socialization opportunities**

   Parents may tend to neglect or over-emphasize this aspect of the child's rehabilitation. Normalizing life patterns should be established as much as possible.

5. **The utilization of support systems, including the practice of networking**

   Because of the sudden, unexpected onset of brain injury, family members are usually not aware of available resources and how to access them. Especially during the early post-injury stages, parents should be encouraged to utilize support systems in order to avoid maladaptive patterns of family isolation (Waaland, 1990). Available support systems can include extended family, friends, school or community service representatives, clergy, and networking with other family survivors. This contact helps to reduce feelings of isolation, self-pity, and the perception that "no one else could understand." Fears, anger, hopes, dreams, and even unacceptable thoughts are often easier to disclose to people who have experienced similar circumstances.

6. **Educational planning during the early stage of re-entry into the family**

   Such planning can be extremely important for the young person's morale and the family's direction. Return to school is a major transition for the young person, but careful planning may minimize some of the family's anxiety over this adjustment. This factor assumes that school officials will be contacted as soon as appropriately possible after the young person's medical condition has begun to stabilize.

7. **A realistic acceptance by the health care team of one's own role, expectations, and needs in working with the young person and family members**

    The health professional has an unusual impact on family members, for they see in this individual a source of hope and an anchor during the troubling adjustment family periods. Service providers should understand how they should respond to the varied family needs, and in what way they can contribute to the medical, educational, and many daily family concerns. For example, helping professionals can assist the family through educating and providing ongoing consultation to school personnel. Establishing a social support system for the young person can facilitate successful academic re-entry. Family members, however, may need help in learning how to confront teacher insensitivity regarding handling the complexities of homework with someone who is brain injured. Many school problems can be anticipated and prevented through scheduling modifications and appropriate programming. Consequently, most families need some assistance in negotiating the educational system.

There is no way to predict consistently eventual "good" or "bad" adjustment because it is a process and not a singular event. But the family should be given the opportunity to maximize all of its areas of functioning. Identifying family strengths that appear to increase positive functioning may be the key to supporting and building family coping resources (Rivara et al., 1996). Each of the above factors, moreover, rarely all occur together, and successful adjustment may take place without all of them.

Interventions

Emerging from many of the issues discussed in this chapter is the demand for appropriate interventions by health professionals and parents toward their children. It is important that family interventions also be directed to increases in self-care in accordance with the young person's development. In their research with family members affected by TBI, Pieper (1991) and Pieper and Singer (1991) identified many effective interventions and categorized them into the following areas:

Communication

Communication between parents and professionals, for example, should be characterized by honest and concrete explanations emphasizing descriptions, not interpretations. When talking with siblings, their developmental level must be considered. Words have different meanings for children at different ages. A sense of time may be perceived differently by a child. For example, "soon" may mean tomorrow to the child, but "not this week" to the adult. Further, communication should be encouraged between the parents of the young person's friends as well as peers regarding the symptoms of brain injury (Miller, 1995).

Expression of feelings

Children of all ages must be given the opportunity to express their feelings. Siblings, as well as the young person with a brain injury, are grieving in their own way over perceived losses. To handle anger and frustration, older and even younger children might be encouraged to release their feelings in constructive ways, such as with drawings or a journal on what is happening in their lives. Younger children might be encouraged to tell a story about a friend in order to express some of their ideas or feelings.

Emotional supports

While parents are indispensable for the life development of their offspring, other adults and significant others can also be important resources for their children. These adults may also become friends who can share in the emotional support and growth of children. Support also includes available counseling, a descriptive and directive type of intervention which focuses on what is happening here and now and how it can be managed. Groups can be more cost-effective and impactive when providing information and shared, caregiving experiences. However, as with individual counseling, group interventions should be approached cautiously, by carefully exploring the skills of the group leader and the guidelines for confidentiality. Sibling support groups can also be quite helpful since they offer young people an opportunity to express concerns and frustrations and get feedback from others.

Each of these three interventions suggests ways for families to balance their needs, interests, and time. They also can result in a balance between medical management, quality of life, and developmental demands of the child and adolescent (Miller, 1995). Adjusting to a brain injury is a special challenge for a family, requiring the qualities of flexibility, openness, generosity, and the ability to listen to family members. Communication skills and the willingness to allow family members to appropriately express their feelings and take advantage of available support systems are all possible approaches to assist the family in readjusting on a daily basis to the demands of living with a head injury.

Conclusion

For family members, educators, and health professionals, it is important to address psychosocial adjustment issues early in the recovery process of children with brain injury. Solving the continued neurobehavioral difficulties that impact on the family requires an understanding of the complex needs of the young person with a brain injury and the many ways in which TBI can be managed. However, an important theme in this chapter is the emphasis on adaptive outcomes. These are goals which result from both the strengths of families and the awareness by parents and health professionals that families can survive and even have enriching lives while coping with head injury effects. Neurobehavioral problems are a family matter, and good outcomes after brain injury have as much to do with family as they do with the individual child (Patrick and Hostler, 1998).

Personal statement

Celia, a parent's burden

My daughter was 11 years old when she was suddenly hit by a car while riding her bicycle on a street near our home. It was a hit-and-run accident, the car sideswiped Celia, knocked her off the bicycle, and then sped away. That was almost 3 years ago, and since then the lives of the family have been changed.

Celia was unconscious for about 2 hours, and had several facial lacerations and broken ribs. The face and ribs have healed, leaving few scars, but it is her brain injury that has caused us the most family suffering. Unfortunately, Celia was not wearing her helmet; she had dashed off the porch where she'd been sitting when a friend waved to her to ride with her. When she woke up in the hospital the doctor stated that he thought it was just a concussion and that she would be fine in a couple of months. But that is not what happened.

When our daughter came home after 3 days in the hospital, we noticed slight behavioral changes which became more noticeable over time. Normally a very focused, determined child, Celia became easily distracted, quick to lose her temper, and frequently agitated during the day. Though the accident happened during the summer, Celia was involved in a reading program by the local library. Before the accident, she would love to tell us the stories she had read; now she couldn't remember any of the stories immediately after reading them. Finally, we took her to our family physician, who referred us to a pediatric neurologist. He diagnosed a closed head injury caused by the accident and recommended different treatments focusing on behavioral and cognitive goals.

Much to Celia's anger and disappointment, we decided to keep her out of school for a year after my husband and I realized that the school was not equipped to deal with the combination of behavioral and mind problems. So we went the home-study route, with different therapists helping us with the many problems that kept coming our way.

Has the injury made a difference in our family life? It sure has. Both my husband and I, married now for 19 years, are from Ireland. We met here while I was working as a nanny for a wealthy family and Michael was going to school to become a chemist. Now he has a very good job with the federal government, and when our second child was born, I left my job in the embroidery factory and decided to be a full-time homemaker. Celia is the youngest of our four children and the only girl. Our oldest just graduated from high school, and the other two boys are in a public high school. Unfortunately, my husband is developing a drinking problem, claiming that he is so terribly upset at what has happened to his only daughter and what kind of a future she will have. Celia is back in regular school in the sixth grade, but has a learning disability and struggles with all of her school subjects. Before the accident she was the brightest person in the class. It is now a disappointment, a cloud that we have to live with every day.

Celia's injury has caused problems, but it has also been a learning experience. Her brothers assume many more responsibilities, like making sure her home and social environment are safe. They have become more vigilant about the welfare of someone else. Perhaps they are closer to each other, if adolescent brothers are able to be close with one another. My husband, as I have mentioned, has not been dealing with all of this very well. I have urged him to get help with his drinking, but he says he is not ready and he is mad at God for allowing this to happen to us. Fortunately, he is not abusive to me or the children. I guess you would call him a "silent drinker," preferring to carry his sorrow in private and wall himself off from all of us. He now doesn't do much with the boys, and that is very painful for me.

I think I am managing pretty well. Celia gets frustrated very easily over her schoolwork, has trouble continuing a conversation, and when there is loud noise in the house, she becomes very upset, shouting and yelling at us. A previously quiet girl has become a screamer. But each morning I write down three goals I wish to accomplish for that day, and this provides a structure for my daily life. I am very specific about these goals, and part of this exercise is to identify those stressors in my life. I don't like my friends to tell me what the stressors are. I should know what is bothering me. Also, I meet twice a month with a group of parents who have children who are brain-injured. What a help these people have been. It took awhile to accept the need for this group. I wasn't ready until I realized that I just didn't know what to do about behavior and school problems. The group gives me ideas about how to manage Celia's temper and outbursts and how to deal with my boys, who at times, I know, feel resentful about so much attention that Celia receives from us. These people have also become my friends, and without them the days would be longer and the future might seem really hopeless.

I pray that Celia will learn to manage her difficulties — prayer, support, and competent professional intervention are what we have. But there is something else that I have learned and it is an important part of my dealing with this. I have become an advocate for my daughter, pleading her cause to her teachers and health professionals. I am, by nature, a quiet person, but being shy and unassertive as a parent of a child with a head injury will get me nowhere. First of all, I don't understand much of the information the doctors are communicating to me, and I must speak out if I wish to understand what is going on. The school situation is something else. My daughter needs some classroom accommodations, and if I am lucky, someone may suggest these to me. Otherwise, I have to learn what is needed and then go after it. Then there is the whole issue of discipline. The group I attend has given me some good ideas, but I have to search for people who are experts in behavioral management. I am not a leader — just a person who stands up for the rights of my family and who wishes the best quality of life for our children. And with my advocacy I try to be good to myself. Taking care of yourself is very important. I am not a selfish person, but I look for new activities in which all the family can participate. These new activities bring variety to all of us and give us all some satisfaction. It makes thinking about the unknown future more bearable.

Discussion questions on the personal statement

1. Why is a "hit and run" more complicated for a family to deal with?
2. Was the doctor's statement that "she would be fine" helpful or not?
3. Was the family adequately prepared for the changes, manifested by Celia, when she returned home? If not what could have been done to facilitate the transition?
4. Do you think it was better to keep Celia at home rather than have her attend school? What were some other options?
5. Discuss the issues and implications of a child's gender as related to a family's reaction to a brain injury.
6. How should a family member be approached when substance abuse has become a means of coping with a brain injury and a roadblock to adjustment?
7. Do you think that the adjustment to the brain injury of an "average child" is different from that of a brain injury to a "gifted child"?
8. How are religious beliefs manifested in this personal statement?
9. Do you think that the mother is coping well? Are there areas that should be considered and attended to? In the present? The future?
10. Are there any risks to being an advocate?
11. Discuss how roles in the family have changed as a result of Celia's brain injury.

Set 4. Who should pay for the care of a person with a brain injury?

Perspective

In addition to the emotional and physical complexity surrounding brain injury, families must also deal with complex financial realities.

If insurance is limited or nonexistent or if large settlements are not viable, families are often forced to turn to other sources of support which are limited in scope and impact. At this point, families are forced to re-evaluate the situation, and they are often faced with very difficult choices. Often the choices are not who *should* pay, but who *can* pay, who *wants* to pay, and who *is willing* to help.

Exploration

1. If you were in need of significant financial assistance from your family, would they respond? Why or why not?
2. Would you be available on a long-term basis to provide maximum financial assistance for a member of your family who had a brain injury, spinal cord injury, AIDS, or Alzheimer's Disease?

Set 5. My family and brain trauma: where do we stand?

1. List five ways your family could contribute to the care of a family member with brain injury.
2. If you had a brain injury, would you want *your* family involved in your care? Why or why not?
3. What would be the most difficult aspect of family involvement for you?
4. What has been, is, or would be most difficult for your family in caring for a child who has a brain injury?
5. List the characteristics of your family which help in the care of a loved one.
6. What are the characteristics of your family which hinder the caregiving process?
7. Do you feel that you are fully functioning in your own life so that you are a role model for others?
8. Would this change if you had a brain injury?
9. Which family member would "understand" if you had a brain injury? If you had AIDS?
10. Who would not be able to understand? Why?
11. Who in your family would be least able to cope with or adapt to illness? To brain injury?
12. Can brain injury be prevented?
13. If brain injury can be prevented, why does it occur?
14. Would you be in favor of placing a limit on financial awards in brain injury cases?
15. Should lawyers be limited to a 6% "commission" on all personal injury cases?
16. What is your position on sharing large awards with persons who were brain injured by an uninsured motorist who had no financial resources?
17. What are the benefits of a 5 million dollar settlement in a brain injury case?
18. What are the liabilities of a 5 million dollar settlement for the injured person and his or her family?

19. Does the state have the right to mandate the use of seatbelts and motorcycle helmets? If a person is brain injured and not wearing them, should his or her insurance be reduced? Cancelled?
20. Write a question that has not been asked that would be most important and relevant to your family's adaptation, coping, and survival of the brain injury experience.

References

Barrett, K. (1999) Psychiatric sequelae of brain injury in children and adolescents, *Curr. Opin. Psychiatr.*, 4, 405–408.

Camplair, P.S., Kreutzer, J.S., and Doherty, K.R. (1990) Family outcome following adult traumatic brain injury, in *Community Integration Following Traumatic Brain Injury*, Kreutzer, J.S. and Wehman, P., Eds., Paul H. Brookes Publishing Company, Baltimore, 207–221.

Clark, E. (1996) Children and adolescents with traumatic brain injury: reintegration challenges in educational settings, *J. of Learning Disabil.*, 29(5), 549–551.

Clark, E., Russman, S., and Orme, S. (1999) Traumatic brain injury: effects on school functioning and intervention strategies, *School Psychol. Rev.*, 2, 242–250.

Coppa, C., Hepburn, J., Strauss, D., and Yody, B. (1999) Return to home after acquired brain injury: is the family ready?, *Brain Injury Source*, 3, 18–21.

Donders, J. and Ballard, E. (1996) Psychological adjustment characteristics of children before and after moderate to severe traumatic brain injury, *J. of Head Trauma Rehabil.*, 11, 7–14.

Guthrie, E., Mast, J., and Richards, P. (1999) Traumatic brain injury in children and adolescents, *Child Add. Psych.*, 4, 807–815.

Hux, K. and Hacksley, C. (1996) Mild traumatic brain injury: facilitating school success, *Intervention in Sch. And Clin.*, 31(3), 158–166.

Kehle, T.J. and Clark, E. (1996) Interventions for students with traumatic brain injury: managing behavioral disturbances, *J. of Learning Disabil.*, 29(6), 633–643.

Kraus, J.F., Rock, A., Hemyari, P. (1990) Brain injuries among infants, adolescents, and young adults, *Am. J. of Disabl. Child.*, 144, 684–691.

Lazar, M. and Menaldino, S. (1995) Cognitive outcome and behavioral adjustment in children following traumatic brain injury, *J. of Head Trauma Rehabil.*, 10, 55–673.

MacFarlene, M.M. (1999) Treating brain-injured clients and their families, *Family Therapy*, 26, 13–30.

Michaud, L., Rivara, F., Jaffe, K., Fay, G., and Dailey, J. (1993) Traumatic brain injury as a risk factor for behavioral disorders in children, *Arch. Of Phys. Med. And Rehabil.*, 74, 368–375.

Miller, B. (1995), Promoting healthy function and development in chronically ill children: a primary care approach, *Fam. Syst. Med.*, 13, 187–200.

Patrick, P.D. and Hostler, S.L. (1998) Neurobehavioral outcomes after acquired brain injury in childhood, *Brain Injury Source*, 2, 26–31.

Patterson, J.M. (1988) Chronic illness in children and the impact on families, in *Chronic Illness and Disability*, Chilman, C.S., Nunnally, E.W., and Cox, F.M., Eds., Sage Publications, Newbury Park, CA, 69–107.

Pieper, B. (1991) In Home Family Supports: What Families of Youngsters with Traumatic Brain Injury Really Need, New York Head Injury Association, Albany, NY.

Pieper, B. and Singer, G. (1991) Model Family Partnerships for Interventions in Children with Traumatic Brain Injury, New York State Head Injury Association, Albany, NY, 15 pp.

Rivara, J.M., Jaffe, K.M., Polissar, N.L., Fay, G.S., Liao, S., and Martin, K.M. (1996) Predictors of family functioning and change 3 years after traumatic brain injury in children, *Arch. Phys. Med. and Rehabil.*, 77, 754–764.

Rosenthal, M., Christensen, B.K., and Ross, T.P. (1988) Depression following traumatic brain injury, *Arch. Phys. Med. And Rehabil.*, 79, 90–103.

Waaland, P.K. (1990) Family response to childhood traumatic brain injury, in *Community Integration Following Traumatic Brain Injury*, Kreutzer, J.S. and Wehman, P., Eds., Paul H. Brookes Publishing Company, Baltimore, 235–248.

Wade, S., Taylor, H., and Drotar, D. (1998) Family burden and adaptation during the initial year after traumatic brain injury in children, *Pediatrics*, 1, 110-116.

chapter three

Impact of brain injury on the adult

A brain injury can be as damaging to the personality as it is to the body. Personality and emotional changes are the most difficult aspects of post injury adjustment (Rosenthal et al., 1998). In fact, brain injury is quite different from most other conditions that cause dependency because injury to the brain is often more pervasive in its effects. Frequently, there are limitations in mobility, cognitive ability, emotional stability, and other functional capacities (Anderson and Parente, 1985; Bergland and Thomas, 1991; DeJong et al., 1990; Varney and Menefee, 1993). The effects of brain injury, such as difficulties with self-awareness, self-regulation, fluency of expression of thoughts and feelings, and inhibition of emotions can persist beyond the recovery period and often result in long-term personality changes, sometimes affecting the ability to function in relationships (Armstrong, 1991; Kaplan, 1993). Lezak (1986) believes that many persons with brain injury have limited awareness of how much they have changed, and their greatest handicaps flow from impaired capacities for control, regulation, and adaptation of complex behavior.

Without first understanding the complex psychosocial problems related to the total brain injury experience, the interactions of limitations make the task of effectively working with adults living with brain injury difficult. The individual with brain injury is usually attempting to manage the various emotional and cognitive changes, and while doing so creates other changes in his family, including a new meaning for family life (Morton and Wehman, 1995). If a person is continually angry about his limitations, for example, then the anger will frequently be projected onto others, creating an atmosphere of tension and anxiety. A brain-injured family member who refuses to participate in prescribed therapies, claiming, "I don't have a problem with that," will cause frustration and disappointment within the family. The lingering presence of these emotions can inhibit the family from assisting their family member to achieve stabilizing rehabilitation goals. Optimum intervention, treatment, and rehabilitation require not only sound medical information, but also an awareness of the effects of the brain injury on the person with the injury and the family lifestyle (Antonak et al., 1993; Kerr, 1977; Livneh and Sherwood, 1991; Vash, 1981). This chapter will focus on the consequences of brain injury on the person who has experienced the trauma.

Some determinants of a person's psychosocial reaction to a brain injury

Brain injury can be caused by a number of physical problems: trauma, anoxia, ruptured aneurysm, or brain abscess. Only in recent years have many persons been surviving the initial medical events which produce residual brain damage (MacFarlene, 1999). This increased survival rate has facilitated the emergence of new treatment approaches, many of which emphasize the productive functioning of the total person after the injury although adult survivors have unique problems. An understanding of emotional factors can play a key role in this functioning, but basic to this awareness is a knowledge of why the person with brain injury is reacting in such a way. Note, however, that such reactions are not static, but more developmental. In other words, an individual with brain injury may show specific reactions because of certain stages in the recovery and rehabilitation process. After discharge from in-hospital rehabilitation care, for example, a person may display enthusiastic hope for complete recovery and denial of any long-term limitations. In another phase of recovery beginning after 6 months, the individual may act irresponsibly and irritably and he may be self-centered. At a later time, such as 15 months or longer after hospitalization, the person may become a difficult, childlike dependent family member (Lezak, 1986). As the expectation of full recovery by a person with severe impairment becomes less and less realistic over time, a specific emotion or combination of emotions may dominate this individual's behavior, such as depression, performance anxiety, defensiveness, and confusion. A lingering hope may later give way to angry outbursts with the gradual acknowledgment that certain brain injury effects will probably be permanent. Besides specific recovery stages, there are other determinants to a person's reaction to brain injury, some of which are:

1. **Severity and type of traumatic brain injury:** Emotional withdrawal from family and friends and affective disturbances such as radical mood swings and depression can be caused by the severity of the injury. There is a lack of confirmatory evidence for the assertion that the severity of the injury is definitely linked to specific emotional and behavioral changes in individuals experiencing brain trauma (Boake and High, 1996; O'Shanick, 1998). Families of individuals with severe traumatic brain injury (TBI), however, still report that personality changes are their most significant concerns (Morton and Wehman, 1995).
2. **The personality makeup of the individual before brain injury:** If a person is accustomed to being dependent on others for most daily needs and has always been reluctant to show initiative or independent

behavior, that person may react to a brain injury by becoming even more dependent than before the injury onset. If a person views himself exclusively as a vigorous, sexually active, and physically strong individual, a brain injury may cause heightened feelings of depression. Other factors included in one's personality makeup prior to brain injury are self-esteem, motivation, emotional needs, and vulnerability. If before the onset of injury an individual has experienced many losses or severe illness, has achieved academically and socially only with the greatest effort, has had other physical or mental handicaps, or there is the presence of other serious illnesses in the family — especially another person who has had a brain injury — the individual with the current brain injury might be depressed and choose poor coping strategies (Christ and Adams, 1984; Rosenthal et al., 1998). At the same time, these previous experiences might have assisted the person in learning more positive ways to adapt to this new loss. If, pre-injury, an individual had the continued satisfaction of competence in handling many life tasks, and his emotional needs have been achieved, feelings of adequacy may return gradually during post-trauma. However, due to a depletion of resources, coping with a prior crisis does not mean that the person can deal with a new and unique experience such as brain injury.

3. **Body image and related factors:** These include the type of symptoms, whether they are disabling or in a body region that carries special importance, whether the brain injury is closed or open, and the severity of the injury (Livingston and Brooks, 1988). For example, since a brain injury may affect memory, this could be uniquely devastating to a lawyer. Similarly, if an athlete's motor ability is affected, it could mean loss of career. An open brain injury may leave disfigurement which, in turn, may stimulate negative attitudes toward the injured person.

4. **The person's previous satisfaction with selected activities:** While a brain injury frequently causes decreased memory, if a person can recall during post-injury those satisfactions with paid employment, leisure, marital, or household activity these memories can provide a sense of satisfaction. This, in turn, can stimulate hope and optimism during the recovery period. The depression, which lingers with many brain-injured persons, can often be minimized with these moments of recall and the temporary conviction that such satisfactions may be regained. The real loss consequent to brain injury is that the pervading limitations resulting from the injury may preclude a person from maintaining a job and selected activities and thus may necessitate learning new skills. Such a learning process may be a unique challenge.

5. **Presence or absence of therapeutic intervention:** Appropriate early intervention could help someone to focus more on the residual assets than the limitations of brain injury, and this perspective could help to minimize a lingering depression, as well as facilitate an aggressive attitude of coping rather than wishing brain injury did not exist. It is

not only the process of early intervention, however, which can make a difference in a person's emotional reaction. The attitudes of health professionals and how they communicate information about brain injury when providing treatment and rehabilitation can also have a decided impact on an individual. A physician or nurse who only emphasizes what one cannot do instead of what one's residual capabilities are may be inadvertently undermining that person's hope.

6. **Familial and societal reactions to brain injury:** Family members can have a profound influence on how an individual will react to his or her brain injury. Because of a brain injury, roles within the family system are quickly and often permanently changed (MacFarlene, 1999). Economic and relationship changes also occur, as well as the family changes resulting from dealing with unpredictable behavior. Issues of blame, consequently, often surface in the family system, and when the person with a brain injury perceives these changes, guilt feelings accompanied by frustration and depression are frequently developed. A person with brain injury also faces familial inconsistency, social injustice, and mixed attitudes from the family. Increased tensions and discord in family and marital relationships during the post-acute phase of recovery may influence the emotional response and coping styles of the person with head injury (Rosenthal et al., 1998). Stereotypical ideas about brain injury and unrealistic or negative expectations from family members concerning performance in the home represent a challenge to the person with brain injury and can foster feelings of inadequacy.

7. **Religion and philosophy of life:** For varied reasons, a person may feel that brain injury is a punishment for past sins. They may believe that the acceptance of loss associated with brain injury is an opportunity to meet a physical, as well as spiritual challenge. Drawing from spiritual resources may alleviate feelings of anguish caused by brain injury and encourage hope. This hope may facilitate a more optimistic attitude which focuses on this life as a transition to the next.

8. **The life stage of the person:** People go through many life stages as they develop. The timing of brain injury in the lifecycle is particularly important. Most brain injuries occur in the prime of life, a period when certain interpersonal and occupational tasks should be accomplished. Often someone has just begun a new career. When the injury occurs at a time when a person has great expectations, the emotional reaction could be more severe. For example, a 21-year-old unmarried man or woman living with his or her parents may experience a brain injury at a time when college graduation or a significant job promotion is approaching. The injury precipitates a disruption in life plans, and the awareness of the disruption often facilitates depression and inappropriate behavioral outbursts (Christensen et al., 1994). This disruption can be more complicated if an adult child becomes brain injured, is abandoned by a spouse, and returns home to family.

9. **Ability to live with uncertainty and ambiguity:** While denial of one's limitations caused by a brain injury is a frequently recognized characteristic of individuals with head trauma, the different unpredictable cognitive, physical, and emotional aspects of brain injury during the indefinite post-trauma period can be quite troubling. It may be a long time before achieving symptom stability, and for individuals who are accustomed to having a measure of control over many life events, such as health, career, and family life, living with the unknown and episodic occurrence of symptoms may bring continued anxiety, irritability, and impatience.

10. **Specific location of the brain injury or lesion:** Healthy emotion, reasoning, and goal exploration are dependent on frontal lobe connections with the limbic system, and "emotional reaction is a collaboration between the left and right, superior and inferior areas of the frontal lobe, each of which stimulates and inhibits positive and negative emotions" (Armstrong, 1991, p. 17). Also, depression characterized by anxiety, fear, and sometimes agitated, hostile, or aggressive behavior can occur in right hemisphere dysfunction, while depression characterized by sadness, lethargy, and feelings of perserverance can occur with left hemisphere dysfunction (Von Knorring, 1983).

Psychosocial reaction to brain injury

The uniqueness of each brain injury, with its varied sequelae that causes a wide variety of cognitive, behavioral, physical, and emotional problems, presents a challenge in understanding the person's response to a brain injury experience (O'Hara, 1988). Each emotional reaction will be unique, and the response will be influenced by a selective configuration of determinants. For one person, the emotional response may be greatly determined by such factors as family expectations, pre-trauma job experience, and the extent of damage to brain functions. For another, the response may be influenced by religion, early health care intervention, and one's developmental life stage.

Apart from the uniqueness of individual reactions, there are certain themes that are evident across the lives of individuals living with and recovering from a brain injury.

1. **Denial of the implications of the trauma:** Denial may include minimization of any personal threat, existence of negative emotion, loss of cognitive and/or physical abilities, or the possibility that one will not completely recover. Denial with the person experiencing the effects of brain injury may take the form of denying past abilities or current limitations, pushing oneself too hard, and an unwillingness to give up control, identity, and value in the eyes of self and others (Armstrong, 1991). Deaton (1986) reports that denying past abilities may result in avoidance of grief, failure to participate in rehabilitation, and lack of motivation. Acting as though present status is identical

to pre-injury status may also result in a failure to remediate deficits and alienation of family and friends. Deaton further explains that pushing oneself too hard can cause physical injuries and depression.

Denial can also serve an adaptive purpose for it can allow the individual to maintain a sense of self-esteem, reduce stress, and possibly generate encouragement and hope. Because of denial, the person with a brain injury can control, in so far as the individual has the capacity to do so, his or her perception of the trauma and emotional reaction to it (Matt et al., 1988). All in all, however, although denial may reduce immediate distress, it frequently has a detrimental long-term effect (Watson et al., 1984). If a person does not finally acknowledge the limitations caused by the brain injury, then the recovery process may be slowed considerably, and little remediation of deficits can occur.

2. **Grieving over perceived losses:** For those persons with brain injury, grief is a profound sadness or sorrow due to the significant changes or reduction in such areas as health, independence, sense of control over life, established roles inside the home, sexuality, familiar daily routine, and means of productivity. Family members mourn the person who was there before the trauma. Importantly, grief is so many little deaths along the way of recovery and/or possible adjustment. These deaths continue to occur as the individual realizes that selected life functions may not be restored, and one has to come to terms with the eventual possibility of little return to pre-injury capacities (Lewis, 1983). The grieving may be further characterized by the persistent desire for recovery of lost abilities or the need to express negative feelings because of many losses and the inability to do so (Brown, 1990). The grief is often accompanied by feelings of anger and helplessness, and anger is often directed toward others.

3. **Depression:** Mood disorders are among the most frequent psychiatric disturbances associated with TBI. Depression may be the single most common affective complaint of persons with head trauma several months after injury (Christensen et al., 1994). It has been estimated that the prevalence of depressive disorders among those with brain injury is between 20 to 50% (Jorge et al., 1993; Gomez-Hernadez et al., 1997). Psychosocial factors, moreover, are suggested as causal mechanisms in depression. The caregiver system and the disruption of social relationships can influence the development of depression following the stress of head trauma (Rosenthal et al., 1998). There is a significant loss or decrease in pre-injury social contacts, accompanied by an inability to form new social contacts. It is hard to assume any direction of causality, however, since the loss of previous social contacts may contribute to depression and depression may prompt the decrease in leisure activities, resulting in fewer social contacts (Burton and Wolpe, 1994). Feelings of anger, loneliness, frustration, and disappointment are associated with the depression. The depres-

sion is part of the grieving process, and in this depression, the individual recovering from a head injury will experience, bit by bit, the impact of the varied losses upon his or her life.

4. **Guilt:** Guilt is better understood in the context of interpersonal relationships. For example, family members may often express to the person with a brain injury their beliefs on why the trauma occurred, such as not wearing a seatbelt or a motorcycle helmet. This blaming type of communication often results in feelings of inadequacy, shame, sadness, agitation, self-condemnation, and anger. It may be extremely difficult for the family and significant others to accept the reality of what has happened, and consequently they deal with their feelings by blaming the person for all the changes.

5. **Social isolation:** Though identified as a significant behavior that accompanies depression, decreased social contact and the disruption of friendships post-trauma facilitate a period of social isolation. The change in social contacts can create extreme loneliness and further promote the dependence on the family for social activities and social interaction (Morton and Wehman, 1995).

6. **Coping styles:** Individuals with a brain injury will adapt selected coping mechanisms that represent strategies for dealing with the perceived losses. Denial is a popular coping style among these persons, but coping may also include (1) displacement — anger over what one has lost may be displaced among relatives, friends, or others; (2) regression — reverting to past methods of gaining gratification, as when one formerly self-reliant person becomes extremely dependent; and (3) intellectualization — belief by one, especially if one is older, that, "I have lived a full life ... it could have been much worse ... perhaps I now will become a better person" (Brown, 1990).

   Coping styles include the varied modes of dealing with the challenges ranging from pain, perceived losses, an uncertain future, redirection of goals, and relationship changes. Coping styles can be more problem-focused, such as seeking information and support, or emotion-focused, such as releasing anger or accepting the situation with resignation. These coping styles are constantly changing cognitive and behavioral efforts to manage specific external and internal demands which are viewed as taxing the resources of the person with an illness or disability (Matt et al., 1988). Many coping strategies are really palliative, such as problem-focusing and denial, which allow an individual to maintain self-esteem.

7. **Acceptance:** A recognition of limitations may eventually facilitate an appropriate life adjustment that includes gaining a new perspective on living. Individuals with brain injury may begin to see that their experience does not depend totally on what has been lost and that they may eventually be able to handle even a greatly altered life (Coppa et al., 1999). This acceptance is the mental decision to live with the realities, the deeply ambivalent feelings, and the new mode

of living. New satisfactions or capacities replace, when it is possible, those which have been lost, and old relationships are renegotiated based on new realities; some will be given up and new ones will be formed. It is a gradual process of redefining the self through new interactions based on things as they are now.

Integral to an understanding of a person's reaction to brain injury is attention to the re-socialization process that should occur after the in-hospital phase of brain injury treatment. Cogswell (1968) has written about the re-socialization process with persons who have a spinal cord injury. Often a similar re-socialization may occur with persons who are brain-injured. Namely, during out-patient treatment, the individual will be cautious in the selection of social opportunities, and when possible, he or she will carefully choose settings that have frequently been used, only associating with long-time friends. Because one eventually realizes the extent of physical, cognitive, and emotional limitations, and goes through a period of readjustment of one's perception of self-confidence, remaining abilities, and realistic opportunities, the person with a brain injury may become cautious about involvement in any new life plans, associations, or even career opportunities. Such cautiousness is a reflection of feelings of vulnerability and "being different." On the other hand, a consequence of brain injury could be a very different reaction and the person could replace caution with impulsiveness.

Conclusion

Personality and emotional disruption have a decided impact on the life adjustment of those with brain injury. Such disruption may persist for several years, only contributing to adaptive difficulties. With an understanding of the complexity of brain injury, both the family and the health professional are better able to approach brain injury from a perspective based on hope tempered by reality. From this frame of reference, effective interventions can be designed that may help the person and his family live more adaptively with the realities of brain injury and the other challenges of life and living. The following personal statement, *Homecoming of a Brain-injured Veteran*, by Paul Murphy, presents the impact of brain injury on a person over a 30-year period. It is a sensitive journey through loss, trauma, fulfillment, and attainment, and validates the premise that there can be life after a brain injury.

Personal statement

Homecoming of a brain-injured veteran
by Paul

In 1967, my family was going through a transition. My parents were contemplating a separation, my older brother had recently married, one of my sisters was leaving for nursing school, the other was just beginning high school, and I was entering the Marines. The roles of my family were definitely changing and the family was facing a stressful time. It appeared that the family as I knew it was ending. It was apparent we would no longer be the same. My mother said that with everyone leaving our house, it was too big to manage alone, and she moved into a small two-bedroom apartment with my younger sister. The day before I left for boot camp I helped them settle into their new home. We were all starting over with new lives, fears, dreams, and independence.

I could not wait to go to boot camp, because for the first time in my life I would be on my own. Little did I realize the military allowed little independence. My independence was limited, but to a 17 year old, it was relished. However, that new independence was short lived. Halfway through my tour in Vietnam, I sustained a serious head wound that not only changed my life, but those of the rest of my family.

My home address was my mother's apartment complex, so she was the first to hear of my injury. Through various sources I learned of the events that took place in my absence. My mother was very close with her neighbors and proudly told them all of her son, the Marine, serving in Vietnam. Whenever the postman came they would yell, "Gert, he's here!" and my mother would check the mailbox for a letter from me. One morning in 1968, a Marine officer and a Staff Sergeant showed up at the apartment complex; all who noticed them were anxious with curiosity. This was a bad omen. The telegram they delivered said I had been seriously injured in combat and sustained a head wound, that the prognosis was poor, and further telegrams would keep them advised of any change. My mother was alone when the startling news was delivered and her reaction was that of shock and fear — shock that I was injured and fear that I could still die from my injury. The information in the telegram was minimal and the extent of my injury was not known. She would have to wait for the next telegram for information on any further progress.

The vagueness of the information on my injury brought about questions that would go unanswered for some time which made the wait tormenting. Daily, my family asked the same questions. How injured was I? Would I live, and if I did live, would I be able to function? Foremost in my mother's mind was that I had a brain injury. My mother's experience with head-injured victims was during World War II when most injuries to the head involved blindness. Telegrams began to arrive every day and stated that my condition was slowly improving, but there was still little mention of the actual extent of the injury. Telegrams reassured her that my prognosis was also improving, but questions as to how I would live as a blind person became the focus of my mother's concern, just not knowing was upsetting. She blamed herself for my injury and was laden with guilt because she felt her signature allowed me to enter the Marine Corps in the first place.

Every little bit of information that was received helped lessen the burden my family was carrying and prepared them somewhat for my return, but they were still unsure of what to expect. Due to the extent of my injury, I was unable to be transported to the U.S. for 2 months. This prolonged time furthered the agony and fears my family had. By being left in the dark about my injury, my family grew uneasy, and constant feelings of hopelessness existed. A Red Cross nurse wrote a letter for me, but I was unaware of its ramifications. While the letter let my family know exactly how I was feeling, because I did not write it, it affirmed the notion my mother had that I was blind. She went about rearranging her tiny apartment making it more maneuverable for a blind individual. It was assumed by the family that I would be living with my mother when I returned and that she would care for me. My mother was fearful of the severity of my injury and unsure whether she, alone, could handle caring for me. Other members of the family offered support, but they did not live at home and it appeared that she alone would be caring for me.

When I finally returned to the States I was placed in Chelsea Naval Hospital. I remember my first day back in Massachusetts, lying there in a crowded neurology ward. It wasn't so long ago that I was on a train headed to boot camp in South Carolina. Then, I was filled with feelings of anticipation and excitement about the new life ahead of me. Now I was filled with sad feelings, knowing that adventure was over, and I was fearful of what the future held. My loss had been more than physical; I also had lost my family. I did not know who would be there for me.

The day my mother and brother visited me, I was asleep. They were shocked to see me as an emaciated shell of what I used to be. They were relieved to see that I was not blind, but were upset upon discovering my disability. Fragmentations from a mortar round had penetrated my skull and I was paralyzed on my right side which was the reason for the Red Cross nurse writing my letter. According to the doctors, my damage was so severe that the chances of rejuvenation were very slim. I reassured them I could manage, but they fell over themselves trying to help. I had time to get familiar with my disability, but had difficulty dealing with their unnerving attempts to assist. I feared my future would be living a piteous existence with loved ones who felt they were helping, but were only making it more difficult for me to be independent.

After 6 months at Chelsea Naval Hospital I went home, the only home available. My family had been in turmoil before I entered the military and I feared not having a permanent place to live when I got out of the hospital. I knew I could sleep at my mother's apartment on the couch when I was on leave, but now it was for an undetermined time. Home was my mother's tiny apartment, which was located on the third floor. I felt displaced, my old room and security were gone, and I felt like an intruder. My disability afforded little mobility and the stairs became a barrier. I became a prisoner in a tiny two-bedroom apartment. My mother had to deal with my complaining and progressive seizure disorder. I had daily grand mal seizures and very little medication at that point. Nobody knew what to do, and we grew more tense in an already tense environment. My mother's only solace was weekly shopping trips with my sister-in-law. While I had a lot of moral support, no relief existed.

In spite of continuous tension between me and my mother, I found her support to be a valuable source of strength in dealing with my losses. She encouraged me to seek out new methods where I could express myself. At first I felt she was interfering, but later I realized if I couldn't change my body, I'd change my mind. My younger sister also shared the apartment along with my mother and me. She felt that her privacy was being imposed upon when I returned home. She had difficulty expressing herself to me and pretty much kept her distance. Being deaf and the baby of the family, she was used to getting all the attention, but when I returned that role changed. Having a disability, she was always just a little different from the rest of the family; now I held that role. She tried dealing with my difference, but it was both confusing and frightening to her. Like the rest of my family, she did not understand what was wrong with me. It took her a while to just get used to me being there and invading her former privacy. I was a stranger to her; I was a stranger to my family.

Not long after I was home, my mother became a patient and had to deal with her own loss when she had a mastectomy. It was hard for me to show my depression when my mother was feeling so much pain with her loss. I felt compelled to help her after all the love and support she provided me in my losses. Her strength gave me strength. We provided each other with needed support over our losses and became closer than ever.

The roles of the family had changed drastically in 3 short years. My father held the family purse strings while I was in Vietnam and still managed to control them after I returned. Getting money for food and rent was painfully difficult. Money from the military and the Veterans Administration was long coming and nowhere in sight. It was a daily struggle. The difficulty drew me and my mother together. My mother became less of a mother and more of a friend. We were like two wounded animals living in the same den. We were just scratching out an existence. My father continued to be as uninvolved as possible. He did not live with us and was not affected by the daily traumas. He was not available to lighten the load or to give me and my mother a break from each other. My brother, however, became the significant male in the family, for a short while. He became the muscles in the family doing all the difficult tasks a father would normally do, or else we would do for ourselves. He became the main source of transportation and was depended upon by me and my mother. When there was a difficult task, he was called. This created friction between his wife and my mother. I also felt tension in our relationship. He felt obligated to do for my mother and me and I felt guilty because he did so much. He unwittingly made me more aware of my disability.

My other sister was in nursing school and when she came home she became our source of constant medical questions. At first, she became overwhelmed and refused to answer anything, but after seeing me continuously having seizures she was able to help come up with a good behavioral plan. Her skills and caring saved me from much pain. However, in the beginning it was difficult having her living at home and refusing to help. It took a while, but I was able to listen to my sister and I became a good consumer regarding my medical needs. I felt like an intruder with my disability, imposing upon my mother, brother, and sisters, and at times they made me feel the part. It was difficult for every person involved with me and my change. The family spent a long fearful time not knowing if I would live or die or what condition I was in. They were happy to see me alive, but no longer knew who I was.

Conclusion

The roles of my family prior to the brain injury were vague; we were all changing. After my brain injury, more questions than answers were created. The questions of who would care for me seemed clear in the minds of some people — my mother would be the primary caregiver. No one ever asked her whether or not she wanted the job or even if she was capable. The family members were thankful that I had not died, however, it was hard having to live with a stranger who could be difficult to deal with.

The roles of my family became defined after I returned from Vietnam. While it was not their choice, they were forced to react to my disability. I know it was hard on my family when I came home. We could have used assistance in dealing with the trauma, but we received no professional help. Back in 1968, little was known about head injuries. They were all told I was lucky to be alive and not to expect many changes.

Today, 32 years later, more information exists about brain injuries and the prevention of head injuries, but head injuries still happen. I have learned many lessons with my brain injuries. While no two brain injuries are the same, all brain-injured individuals require certain elements to mend. They need understanding, support, and time. Without any of these elements, no matter how severe the survivor's injuries are, they will have difficulty recovering.

My family provided me with understanding and support. It took time for me to mourn my wounds. While I was able to understand my losses, others may not be able to due to the severity of their injury. What is important is that they are given the time for their brains to mend and support throughout the process by family, friends, and the medical profession to help acknowledge the brain-injured survivor's accomplishments, no matter how small. Most brain injury survivors hold onto yesterday and don't realize their losses. Usually "survivors" state they will get back to what they were before — chances are they never will. In their journey back they need realistic support as to their capabilities. It is a hard lesson to learn when you cannot do what you did before. Recovery for a brain-injured person means living to the best of one's potential.

Discussion questions on the personal statement

1. What would have made Paul's coping with his losses easier?
2. Is it "fair" that he had a brain injury?
3. Could you have done as well as Paul if you were in his situation?
4. What happened to his mother? Was it "fair" that she became the sole caretaker?
5. Do you think he felt responsible for her illness?
6. What approaches would you use to have Paul's father become involved?
7. Is 32 years a long time to be challenged by the effects of a brain injury?
8. What are the issues that should be attended to in the future?
9. How will Paul cope if he sustains another brain injury?
10. Would Paul be prepared to cope better with a spinal cord injury because he has mastered and managed prior losses?
11. What kind of stress would be created if his wife became disabled?
12. If Paul had a child with a disability, how do you think he would cope?
13. How would you have assisted Paul's family to better understand and live with the effects of Paul's brain injury?
14. What were the forces within Paul's support system that enabled him to excel and reach his goals?
15. What does living to the best of one's potential mean for the person and the family living with a brain injury?

Set 6. Brain injury and the family: how would you like to be traumatically brain injured like me?

Perspective

Imagine that you are 24 years old, living in a brain injury rehabilitation facility, and have been abandoned by your family. You are often told to control your anger and get along better with your peers because you frequently become very hostile, and primarily express this during recreation periods. How should you feel? How would you feel?

Exploration

The point of this exercise is to explore some issues faced by a person living with a brain injury and the need to appropriately express anger, frustration, distress, and unhappiness. The challenge for the helping professional is to facilitate the expression of feeling, reduce its negative consequence, and create viable alternatives to counter-balance an often harsh reality.

1. Discuss the need to express anger, frustration, sadness, happiness, and hope.

2. How would you react to the partial loss of memory?
3. How would you try to get out of depression?
4. What are the implications of the loss of memory for you?
5. How would a traumatic brain injury impact your hopes, dreams, and aspirations?
6. Would information on the severity of a brain injury of a family member be helpful or harmful to you and your family?
7. Discuss how hope can be helpful and/or harmful.
8. Would peer group counseling be helpful to you? Why? Why not?
9. What family resources do you have? Could you rely on them?
10. What would be the most difficult implications of TBI for you? For a loved one?
11. Do you believe that miracles are possible even when there is limited optimism regarding physical improvements?
12. How would you spend your life if your future was altered by the occurrence of a brain injury?
13. What would you do if your doctor told you to accept your injury in peace rather than seek out treatment or experimental drugs to "cure" your brain injury?
14. How could your family be more helpful?
15. What do you feel you would need the most if you had severe brain injury?

Personal statement

Life is not fair
by Janet

I always thought that when your plane landed and then taxied to its assigned gate, you were quite safe. I was wrong. Three years ago I was returning from a business trip to the Midwest. After the plane stopped, a passenger in front of me suddenly opened the overhead luggage compartment and his metal luggage carrier fell on my head. I was terribly stunned and was taken by ambulance to the hospital. The doctor told me I had a concussion. I thought I'd get better. When I didn't, I went to see a neurologist. One of the doctors told me that blue collar workers complain of pain while people who work with their heads complain of loss of intellect.

I was soon released from the hospital with a diagnosed brain injury. I was exhausted and confused. I would make nonsensical statements and I couldn't even dial a telephone. I couldn't figure out what was going on, and I kept waiting for the other shoe to drop because I knew I wasn't functioning. I was a 43-year-old lawyer who had a great job with a state government. I was unable to use my word processor, and I couldn't make decisions. When I interviewed people, I had trouble figuring out the appropriate questions to ask. Work was a disaster, yet I didn't understand why I was having so much trouble. I thought I just got hit in the head and I didn't understand why the problem wouldn't go away. I was scared that I had Alzheimer's Disease. I couldn't believe that a bump on the head could do all of this. But I stayed at work for a year and a half until they put me on medical disability.

In the past, I dealt very well with personal disasters and illness. My sister died of a brain tumor at age 26. My father had many strokes until I finally had to put him in a nursing home. My son died, my husband had a heart operation, and four members of my family were killed in an automobile accident. I could look at this brain injury in perspective.

I would rather have lost a limb than my head. It totally changed my life. Nothing every stopped me before. If I wanted to do something, I just went and did it. Now, I can't even go to the store and buy a dress or look at a menu and figure out what I should eat. It still hurts that I can't do what I want. I know I can't go back to being an attorney; my personality has changed; I am more short-tempered.

My husband is very supportive. He is a radiologist and enjoys cooking and food shopping. He is also my best friend and he knows more about my condition than I do. And family for me always comes first. The spouse has to be patient, have a sense of humor, be understanding, and be willing to pitch in without devaluing the person or pointing out the way it was before. So much depends on the relationship one had with one's family before the trauma. If there's a sense of commitment and sharing, somehow it will be sustained.

But my friends give me many moments of anxiety. They don't understand because I look normal and I sound normal, but I'm not quite the same person I was. Even a good friend looking at me will say, "There's nothing really wrong with you." Many of my old friends have dropped me, but I have made new friends who accept me as I am.

Right now I am taking a course at a nearby community college to try and regain my reading skills. Though I was totally out of it, currently I am much improved. I have lost some of my motivation, however, and sometimes I have to push myself to go to cognitive rehabilitation or my classes. But I'm looking for a place where people can offer me something, because not all of my cognitive skills are gone. I think that would be very beneficial. If I could do something on a volunteer basis, that would be very meaningful.

Right now I feel frustration, anger, and disappointment. If I had been put in a hospital with my tongue hanging out and drooling, it would be easier to understand. I've never been one to talk about my problems — everybody has problems. Nobody wants to hear about somebody else's problems. People will say, "Oh, I do that," and I have to keep explaining. It's very difficult and frustrating. I do get hurt by some of my old, close friends of 30-some years' duration. There have been a couple of studies done that show educated people who incur disability. Afterward, to avoid the constant explaining and constant devaluing, they seek their own people, not only supportive people but those within their own community who have similar needs. However, I have not done that. I don't believe in sitting and crying my heart out to others. I want to get on with my life. I'd like to find a way of getting out of that box. I haven't as yet.

Discussion questions on the personal statement

1. What are the unique stressors related to a work-related brain injury?
2. Was the doctor's statement about the "blue collar workers" and "people who work with their heads" helpful?
3. What are the unique aspects of being a lawyer with a brain injury?
4. Did Janet receive relevant and helpful information regarding the brain injury recovery process?
5. Did prior family illness have a role in Janet's coping and recovery?
6. Is the loss of friends unusual after a brain injury? If so why?
7. Comment on the importance of the pre-injury family and the marital relationship.
8. What does Janet mean regarding family when she says: "somehow it will be sustained?"
9. Is being told that there is nothing really wrong helpful?
10. What is the most important message Janet is presenting?

References

Anderson, J. and Parente, F. (1985). Training family members to work with the head injured patient, *Cognit. Rehabil.*, July/August, 12–15.

Antonak, R., Livneh, H., and Antonak, C. (1993) A review of research on psychosocial adjustment to impairment in persons with traumatic brain injury, *J. of Head Trauma Rehabil.*, 8, 87–100.

Armstrong, C. (1991) Emotional changes following brain injury: psychological and neurological components of depression, denial and anxiety, *J. of Rehabil.*, April/May/June, 15–22.

Bergland, M.M. and Thomas, K.R. (1991). Psychosocial issues following severe brain injury in adolescence: individual and family perceptions, *Rehabil. Counseling Bull.*, 35(1), 5–22.

Boake, C. and High, W. (1996) Functional outcome from traumatic brain injury: unidimensional or multidimensional?, *Am. J. of Phys. Med. And Rehabil.*, 75, 105–113.

Brown, J.C. (1990) Loss and grief: an overview and guided imagery intervention model, *J. of Ment. Health Counseling*, 12(4), 434–445.

Burton, L. and Wolpe, B. (1994) Depression after head injury: do physical and cognitive sequelae have similar impacts?, *J. Neuro. Rehabil.*, 8, 63–67.

Christ, G. and Adams, M.A. (1984) Therapeutic strategies at psycho-social crisis points in the treatment of childhood cancer, in *Childhood Cancer: Impact on the Family*, Christ, A.E. and Flomenhaff, K., Eds., Plenum Press, New York, 109–130.

Christensen, B., Ross, T., Kotasek, R., Henry, R., and Rosenthal, M. (1994) The role of depression in rehabilitation outcome during acute recovery from traumatic brain injury, *Adv. In Med. Psychotherapy*, 7, 23–28.

Cogswell, B. E. (1968) Self-socialization: re-adjustment of paraplegics in the community, *J. of Rehabil.*, 34, 11–13.

Coppa, C., Hepburn, J., Strauss, D., and Yody, B. (1999) Return to home after acquired brain injury: is the family ready?, *Brain Injury Source*, 3, 18–21.

Deaton, A.V. (1986) Denial in the aftermath of traumatic brain injury: its manifestations, measurement, and treatment, *Rehabil. Psychol.*, 31(4), 231–140.

DeJong, G., Batavia, A.I., and Williams, J.W. (1990) Who is responsible for the lifelong well-being of a person with a brain injury?, *J. of Head Trauma Rehabil.*, 5(1), 9–22.

Gomez-Hernandez, R., Max, J., Kosier, T., Paradiso, S., and Robinson, R. (1997) Social impairment and depression after traumatic brain injury, *Arch. Phys. Med. Rehabil.*, 78, 1321–1326.

Jorge, R., Robinson, R., Starkstein, S., and Arndt, S. (1993) Depression and anxiety following traumatic brain injury, *J. Neuropsychiatr.*, 5(4), 369–374.

Kaplan, S.P. (1993) Five-year tracking of psychosocial changes in people with severe traumatic brain injury, *Rehabil. Counseling Bull.*, 36,(3), 151–159.

Kerr, N. (1977) Understanding the process of adjustment to disability, in *Psychosocial Aspects of Disability*, Stubbins, J. Ed., Springer Publishing Company, New York.

Kreutzer, J. and Sander, A. (1998) Issues in brain injury evaluation and treatment, *Rehabil. Psychol.*, 42, 231–239.

Lewis, K. (1983) Grief in chronic illness and disability, *J. of Rehabil.*, July/Aug/Sept, 8–11.

Lezak, M.D. (1986) Psychological implications of traumatic brain damage for the patient's family, *Rehabil. Psychol.*, 31(4), 241–250.

Livingston, M.G. and Brooks, D.N. (1988) The burden on families of the brain injured: a review, *J. of Head Trauma Rehabil.*, 3(4), 6–15.

Livneh, H. and Sherwood, A. (1991) Application of personality theories and counseling strategies to clients with physical disabilities, *J. of Counseling and Dev.*, 69, 525–538.

MacFarlene, M. (1999) Treating brain-injured clients and their families, *Fam. Ther.*, 26, 13–30.

Marinelli, R.P. and Dell Orto, A.E. (1999) *Psychological and Social Aspects of Physical Disability*, Springer-Verlag, New York.

Matt, D.A., Sementilli, M.E., and Burish, T.G. (1988) Denial as a strategy for coping with cancer, *J. of Ment. Health Counseling*, 10(2), 136–144.

Morton, M. and Wehman, P. (1995) Psychosocial and emotional sequelae of individuals with traumatic brain injury: a literature review and recommendations, *Brain Injury*, 9, 81–92.

O'Hara, C. (1988) Emotional adjustment following minor brain injury, *Cognit. Rehabil.*, March/April, 26–33.

O'Shanick, G. (1998) Personality changes following acquired brain injury, *Brain Injury Source*, 2, 20–23.

Rosenthal, M., Christensen, B., and Ross, T. (1998) Depression following traumatic brain injury, *Arch. Phys. Med. Rehabil.*, 79, 900–103.

Varney, W.R. and Menefee, L. (1993) Psychosocial and executive deficits following closed brain injury: implications for orbital frontal cortex, *J. Head Trauma Rehabil.*, 8(1), 32–44.

Vash, C.L. (1981) *The Psychology of Disability*, Springer Publishing Company, New York.

Von Knorring, L. (1983) Inter-hemispheric EEG difference in affective disorders, in *Laterality and Psychopathology*, Flor-Henry, J. and Gruzelier, R., Eds., Elsevier Science Publishers, New York.

Watson, M., Green, S., Blake, S., and Schrapnell, K. (1984) Reaction to a diagnosis of breast cancer: relationship between denial, delay, and rates of psychological morbidity, *Cancer*, 53, 2008–2012.

chapter four

Impact of brain injury on the family

The brain injury of a family member challenges the core values and resources of the family system. It also has a long-term negative impact on the family. Not only must the family adapt to the emerging needs of persons with brain injuries but it must also continue to maintain a sense of unity by regrouping its members, refocusing its resources, and redefining its functions. How the family reorganizes often depends upon its emotional response to the loss, stress, hope, and reality consequent to the brain injury (Cavallo et al., 1992; Jacobs et al., 1986; McKinlay and Hickox, 1988; Orsillo et al., 1991; Rosenthal and Young, 1988; Williams and Kay, 1991; Zarski et al., 1988; Kosciulek, 1994; MacFarlene, 1999).

This chapter explores how family members react to the complexities of the brain injury experience. Bringing these reactive patterns into sharper focus can enhance the understanding of the influences the family can have on the stabilization of the person with the brain injury. Family members, for example, who deny the existence of a brain injury or its complexity, are not going to effectively assist the patient during the treatment and rehabilitation process. At the same time, a family that has adapted to the implications and reality of brain injury could be a constructive force in the person's life. However, since each family is unique and changing, so are the family reactions to the brain injury of a family member.

Determinants of family reaction to brain injury

There are many causes for the family's reactions to illness and disability in general and brain injury in particular. These factors may not only indicate why a family is reacting in a particular way, but what may be done by health care professionals and other support systems to assist the family in adjusting to a complex, demanding, and changing reality.

Previous history

Family history includes the mental and physical health of the family members, as well as how the family has dealt with previous crises (Rolland, 1994). A chronic, physical illness may seriously hamper the expression of energy required for most caregiving efforts. If a family member has a past history of a mental illness, the family experience of living with the adjustment demands of a head trauma may only trigger memories of painful and unpleasant times, even though the mental illness is now managed. Also, when a life crisis represents an unfamiliar event, the family will usually display confusion and have a more difficult time focusing its resources. When previous crises have identified family resources, and helped to establish coping patterns, then the impact of the disability may be less devastating. Shock and a feeling of helplessness will still be present after the initial diagnosis, but these reactions may be managed more readily if the family has successfully managed other losses. A family whose breadwinner has been out of work for many months because of a severe illness, for example, has had an opportunity to assess its resources as well as expand them. If another member of the family is diagnosed with a severe illness a few years later, the family will often adapt successfully if its resources were used effectively during the previous illness. If coping patterns have been effective in the past, then they will usually be adopted again in the new crisis. However, past success should be considered in the context of the families' inability to deal with a new stressor such as brain injury because their resources have not been replenished and new skills have not been developed relevant to the unique aspects of a brain injury.

The meaning brain injury has to the family

How the family understands brain injury will depend on the kind of information that has been imparted to family members, when and how it was given, and the ability of family members to hear, understand, and believe what is being said. Early and appropriate communication of information by health care professionals and significant others will generally diminish anxiety and allow the family to start working toward adjustment goals. This communication may change the family's understanding of the brain injury impairment. A change in understanding can create higher expectations for the eventual adjustment of the family member. If the family is in doubt about the nature of a brain injury and its implications for the injured family member, this uncertainty will create continued family tension and inhibit the formulation of realistic goals. While information can be helpful, the complex long-term nature of a severe brain injury can also create distress and precipitate a family crisis if family needs are in direct conflict with reality.

Family interaction

The family system that is nurturing, well structured, and has effective communication usually has the potential to develop effective coping mechanisms. In contrast, members of a family system that is indecisive and has contradictory types of behavior will generally act in isolation from one another and have a difficult time reaching out to each other for mutual support. The brain injury experience for this family will usually bring protracted periods of confusion and avoidance behavior in confronting the realistic implications of the brain injury.

Coping resources/family capabilities

Coping resources include various emotional strengths which family members may possess to deal with brain injury. Satisfying work activity, support from extended family, availability of necessary community resources, anticipation of planned activities, and self-help groups can be helpful in times of the continued stress associated with the brain injury experience. Included in these resources are financial means and the ability of family members to use community agencies. A family that has financial protection and will not suffer severe economic hardship because of the brain injury will theoretically cope much better than one for whom brain injury represents a financial disaster. However, some financially secure families have become emotionally bankrupt while poorer families have not only survived but have become emotionally rich. Given the astronomical costs associated with brain injury care, few families can feel that they are completely financially secure and insulated from the long-term issues related to lifetime care.

Who is ill and the status and role of the ill family member with a brain injury

It may make more of a difference to the family if the wage earner or a child is seriously affected by brain injury. For example, if the wife or husband is the major breadwinner and he or she is suddenly brain injured, this could have a decided impact on overall family economic functioning. However, a brain injury to a child can easily result in intense stress if the parents are unable to help each other during the acute stages of adjustment.

The stage of the family lifecycle

Each family stage brings the necessity of accomplishing certain tasks (i.e., raising children or building financial security for the family). The presence of brain injury has a unique impact on the family if the children have left home, and the parents have been planning for their retirement years. Suddenly they are looking at nursing homes or coma management facilities rather than retirement homes.

Nature of pre-injury relationship to the injured person

The family members' perceptions of their relationship to the person with brain trauma are critical components in how the family will adjust. If they perceive the injured family member prior to trauma onset as an energetic contributor to family life, their adjustment to the injury may be characterized by lingering feelings of loss, a reluctance to accept significant differences in the injured family member, and even a false hope that pre-injury functioning will be quickly restored. When family members believe that the person was problematic before the trauma, this conviction will accompany their acceptance of cognitive and behavioral changes after the brain injury event.

Available support systems to the family

Support systems are defined as continuing social aggregates (namely, continuing interactions with another individual, network, group, or organization) which provide individuals with opportunities for feedback of themselves and validation of their expectations of others (Caplan, 1976). The availability of an extended family, support group, or similar resource can make a difference in how a family copes with a brain injury experience. These resources may provide respite care, nurturance, and feelings of acceptance to the family that conveys that despite of what has happened each family member is a worthwhile human being.

The cultural background of the family

The family's culture makes a difference in the member's adjustment to the disability. African-American families, for example, are organized around extended kinship networks that may include blood and non-related persons. Family roles, responsibilities, and functions are often interchanged among family members, a sharing which cuts across generations and gender roles (Carter and Cook, 1991; Cavallo and Savcedo, 1995). There is variability among Latin American families with regard to ethnicity, as in Puerto Rican, Cuban, and Mexican, as well as class differences. Traditional cultural values of fatalism, respect, spirituality, and personalism may often be reflected in the Latino adjustment to a disability event (Dillard, 1983). Within Asian families, moreover, transgenerational beliefs on coping with illness can be particularly important. The concept of obligation is also central in Asian cultures and families, and family obligations, such as providing care for a disabled family member, are indirectly communicated using non-confrontational strategies (Carter and Cook, 1991). In other words, all families have distinctive cultural values and the impact of these values on the characteristics of disability and/or illness adjustment should be recognized.

The issues of blame and guilt within families because of brain injury

The factors of blame and guilt can be strong undercurrents for family members regardless of the cause of the injury. The perception of personal responsibility for the cause of a brain injury can be a strong determinant in family member adaptation. If the brain injured takes responsibility for engaging in the behavior that caused the accident, such as alcohol consumption or not wearing a seatbelt, other family members may adapt more easily to post-injury adjustment demands. Other family members may then feel less guilty. Even with this assumption of personal responsibility, family communications may be blame-laden or used as ammunition in family power struggles.

Nature of family stressors

With brain injury, physical and cognitive impairments are usually perceived by family members as the most stressful. Included among family stressors are family finances, lack of respite care, limited living arrangements, continued anger in the family over undefined issues, and the special needs of the brain injured.

If the health care professional understands the reasons why the family members are responding in a certain way to brain injury, this awareness can form the basis for intervention. For example, when the health professional learns that the family has inadequate knowledge about brain injury, are emotionally receptive to further understanding, and could profit from this communication, intervention efforts might impart information based on facts and convey hope.

Patterns of family reaction to chronic illness

Historically, there have been contributions from researchers on family reactive patterns to long-term illness (Bray, 1977; Christopherson, 1962; Epperson, 1977; Giacquinta, 1977). These models are usually more appropriate when there are clear phases or steps in disability progression and when the end result is more or less predictable. Developmental stage models have been proposed to conceptualize the family's adjustment to severe head injury (Rape et al., 1992). Armstrong (1991) believes that family reactions to traumatic brain injury (TBI) are likely to follow a developmental course, beginning with a response to acute stress which is reactive and crisis-oriented. Lezak (1986) and Romano (1974) developed models to explain a progression of family reactions, with Lezak emphasizing six stages of family adjustment to brain injury, each characterized by distinct perceptions of the patient, expectations for recovery, and family reactions. These reactions by the family range from thankfulness for the patient's survival, anticipation for a full recovery within the first year, and confusion and anxiety as physical recovery begins to slow down, to perceptions of the patient as difficult and dependent, a view accompanied by diminished expectations for improvement (Waaland and Kreutzer, 1988). Romano (1974) believed that families often have unrealistic expectations for recovery and rely heavily on denial, particularly during the early post-injury period. Rocchio (1998) identified three common reactions:

1. Complete recovery was fantasized by family members.
2. Denial caused physical impairments to be ignored or explained away.
3. Inappropriate behaviors were ignored, such as temper tantrums and deviant sexual behavior, and the family was unable to establish limits.

Family reactive models to illness and/or disability may be less useful when the family situation is composed of a multitude of physical and/or emotional problems that have a much more indefinite course. However, families may not adapt to members who are brain-injured, going through a series of distinct, identifiable stages (Rape et al., 1992). Just like brain injuries are so unique that no two individuals will exhibit exactly the same symptoms (Howell, 1978), so too the reaction of family members will be different. There is also an episodic loss reaction by family members to brain injury (Williams and Kay, 1991). The injured family member appears to be improving, family hopes are then increased, and then, unpredictably, there is a cognitive or physical setback, causing a renewed grief reaction among family members.

Within each family attempting to adjust to brain injury, it is not unusual for husbands, wives, and siblings to respond in very different ways. Grieving patterns may also be diametrically opposed, making it very difficult for family members to support and understand one another. Acceptance of the injury, consequently, may mean a realistic assessment and understanding of the significance and long-term effect of losses (Mitiguy, 1990). He explains:

> Instead of an iron door, a thick but transparent curtain
> in the form of coma or disorientation descends be-
> tween family members and the injured person. Their
> grief is suspended as they wait in hope for the curtain
> to lift and, later, for the patient to return to his former
> self (pp. 2–3).

Following the determinants of the family's emotional reaction to brain trauma, developmental stage models have been identified as an important approach to understanding family reactions. But these models do not provide any information on why some families manage to adapt while others become entrenched in a posture of resistance to change (Rape et al., 1992). If the family is viewed as an internally dynamic group of individuals, family members will exhibit differential adaptation patterns following the trauma. It is more appropriate, consequently, to identify reactive themes which may be more applicable to one family member than another.

Themes

Shock

The onset of a traumatic brain event has a sudden, unexpected, and usually extensive effect on the life of family members. Feelings of helplessness, numbness, being overwhelmed, confusion, and perhaps even the temporary loss of self-control result from the initial event. At this time family members need to feel they have hope and that hospital personnel care about the patient.

Denial

With little information or understanding as to what extent the patient will be impaired, family members may deny any implications of the trauma regarding permanent physical, emotional, or intellectual limitations. Denial may also take the form of insistence that the recovery be complete, divine intervention will occur, and minimal future changes to family life will occur. At this time, the denial may serve a positive purpose. Entertaining hopes may give family members the time and opportunity to identify and organize their coping resources.

Grief

Grief is a persistent feeling in families, an emotion resulting not only from the realities of family disruption but from the loss of a family partner with whom family members had a mutual and caring relationship. All of a sudden it becomes a one-way relationship and they miss the person who cared about them in a special way (Mitiguy, 1990). In fact, grief may be especially poignant for the injured person's spouse since the essential loss of a partner is mourned. This mourning is borne alone because society neither recognizes the grief nor provides the support and comfort that usually surrounds those bereaved (Zeigler, 1987). Family grief continues because family members remain in an uncertain state; they're waiting for full recovery but realizing that they may be dealing with the patient's impairments for the rest of their lives.

Gradual realization

As family members become aware that their injured family member is not going to be the same physically, emotionally, and/or intellectually as before the trauma, issues of blame, guilt, anger, and depression emerge. Sibling responses may include withdrawal, hostility, sleeping problems, emotional outbursts, increased rebelliousness, and verbalized resentment (Mitiguy, 1990). During this time family members need questions answered honestly and explanations given in understandable terms (Mathis, 1984). They may also need to learn how to interact with physicians and other health personnel in order to gain needed information and combat feelings of powerlessness.

Reorientation

With the family's slow acknowledgment that the effects of the brain injury will be permanent, individual family members will gradually adjust their life to meet caregiving demands, role reallocation tasks, and perhaps family finance changes. Although grieving can take on a chronic nature, many families do eventually work through feelings of denial, optimism, anger, and depression to a degree of adjustment. For some, this can take several years with varying amounts of time for family members to come to some sense of resolution and acceptance. Yet many families start to educate themselves, seek out supports, assess problems, and plan for the future (Waaland and Kreutzer, 1988). During this period of reorientation, fears about the patient's present and future preoccupy the stressed relatives (Armstrong, 1991; Kreutzer et al., 1994).

This reorientation of personal lives within the context of family life is very difficult for family members. Feelings of blame, anger, and resentment still linger, even accompanied by both a sense of relief that the injured did survive and a conviction of hope that previous functions of the injured will return. During this time of reorientation, the family may attempt to reintegrate the injured person into family life, involving the individual in social activities and household tasks.

As the family engages in their adaptive tasks, and in their understanding that both anger and depression are parts of the grieving process, the physical, personal, social, familial, vocational, and economic ramifications of the disability become apparent. Some families may welcome these changes and perceive living with the disability as a means for renewed family togetherness. Other families may view the necessary changes as manageable and they may believe that their adjustment to the disability is an expression of their commitment and endurance, perceiving the family future as unalterably shaped. Still other families may perceive that the changes caused by the injury are catastrophic (Kreuter et al., 1998). They feel the future of the person with brain injury is hopeless, and that family life will now be characterized as troubled and lonely. Keydel (1991), in her study of families undergoing the adjustment process to a young adult, male member with brain injury, refers to these three adaptive stages as success, survival, and submission. Yet it is not to be assumed that these family characteristics are representative of the final stage in the family coping process. Adaptation to the brain injury event is ongoing, and the family's long-term adjustment might be considerably altered as their perceptions of living with the disability change (Keydel, 1991).

There is yet another way to understand the reactions of family members to brain trauma. The extensive range of negative phenomena with caring for persons with brain injury has been called "caregiver burden" (Chwallisz, 1992). The amount of burden a family member experiences can depend on age, gender, coping styles, how one views the situation, and mental health history prior to the trauma. Objective burden is understood as problems encountered by the injured, such as behavior disturbances and environmental changes experienced by the caregiver, i.e., financial strain, change of role or employment status (Allen et al., 1994). Subjective burden is perceived stress, or the amount of psychological strain on family members that is caused by changes in the person with head trauma. Perceived stress, however, is difficult to define precisely. What may be appraised as harmful or threatening to one family member may not be considered as challenging to another. However, personal burdens are realities caused by daily management responsibilities, perceived limits on family opportunities, and perhaps the lack of personal rewards that persons may experience when caring for the injured.

All of the different adaptive themes identified above, as well as the presence of objective and subjective burden, can be illustrated in a sequential manner. The illustration does not negate the possibilities of a recycling of reactive emotions during the recovery process or any behavior lapses, nor does it negate the uniqueness of one family member's reaction.

> Success

Shock > Denial > Gradual Realization > Reorientation   > Survival

> Submission

Integral to understanding the manner in which families react to the brain injury situation is the awareness that family members will utilize different coping mechanisms as they attempt to adjust to living with the injury (Orsillo et al., 1993). Certain varied coping strategies may be used for a period of time only to then be replaced by other mechanisms. Coping strategies are employed to manage stressful demands, ward off threats to family life, and perhaps even to change the situation. Families who appear to adapt well to the brain injury utilize, with other resources, a more cognitive style of coping which expresses a sense of mastery in regard to their circumstances. Mastery can comprise a variety of skills, including those for changing affective reactions to trying circumstances. Consequently, people who seem to adapt well to difficult circumstances are able to assign a meaning to their difficulties, as well as pinpoint the causes of their physical and emotional reactions to events.

With a cognitive style of coping, there are other ways to view the coping strategies of family members. Pearlin and Schooler (1978) have suggested the following three categories that are very relevant to illness, disability, and brain injury:

1. Strategies to change the family situation (stress, anxiety, confusion, and avoidance by family members), caused by illness or disability. These can include seeking advice and information from knowledgeable persons, and tapping one's own individual strengths, such as communication skills and ability to identify valuable community resources.
2. Strategies to control, not change, family disruptions, anxieties, uncertainties for the future, and feelings of grief and loss. These strategies include positive comparisons formulated by family members (We could be worse off ...), entertaining beliefs that the patient will improve somewhat or that support for caregiving responsibilities is available, utilizing tension reduction approaches, such as relaxation training or pursuing recreational activities, and accumulating knowledge.
3. Strategies to minimize personal discomforts caused by the reality of disability, such as stress, fear, frustration, disappointment, and future uncertainties. These strategies include ventilation, or talking with others about one's problems, distracting oneself with activities, stoically accepting the situation, and even wishful thinking, namely, imagining that someday the family situation will be better. For many family members' prayers can also be an invaluable help to minimize feelings of grief and loss.

The coping strategies used by family members will generally depend on how the individual family member appraises the situation of living with brain injury and one's perception of the resources available. An individual makes a series of judgments concerning the potential effects of events on their emotional wellbeing. In other words, coping involves not only behavior but also varied thoughts on how best to deal with the situation.

The following personal statement, *Almost a Vegetable, by a survivor, mother, and father,* explores the impact of a brain injury from varied perspectives. During the difficult journey to stabilization and rehabilitation, each person drew upon his or her own unique resources and perceptions of the experience.

Personal statement

Almost a vegetable
by a survivor, mother, and father

Changing from a fully functioning young, athletic college student to a comatose, nonverbal invalid can take place in a matter of seconds. Recovery may require years; some may never recover. For me, being alive is a miracle. Following the motorcycle accident that resulted in a brain injury, my family was informed that it was unlikely that I would live. The following presentation is my perspective on my struggle to beat the odds. Not only was I able to win, but I was also able to rise above the physical and emotional strain placed on my life.

As a college student, I was at the point in my life where I had everything going for me. I was happy as a university student, had a girlfriend, and was actively involved as a member of the track team. My preoccupations at that time centered around my independence, future, friends, and the variety of other joys and pleasures which were part of my life.

The summer prior to my senior year I was employed as a construction worker. To reduce the amount of time I would have to spend traveling to my home, I lived in a tent. It was a taste of the pioneer life, living in the outdoors, working and basically enjoying my sense of independence from my family. This need for independence and self-sufficiency had been an issue in the relationship with my parents and had caused some conflict between us. At this time I had no idea that I would soon become the most helpless, dependent person imaginable.

That summer I was riding my motorcycle, enjoying the beauty of a summer's evening. My last recollection was losing control. The next thing I knew it was November and I was in a hospital. Having no speech and partial paralysis, my life at that time was one of confusion, desperation, and challenge. I had a hard time putting the pieces together, but I somehow realized that I was hurting. I knew that I needed people to maintain my life supports since I could not do anything on my own. I decided that if I were to survive, I would have to draw people to me. I could not act up because I would drive them away.

What a difference the support of my family and friends made. They were always there. Their presence and encouragement made me want to make an effort to do as much for myself as others had hoped for me.

Being unable to speak after I came out of my coma, I had to deal internally with the many issues that I was terrified and uncertain of. I wondered, will I ever be able to speak, walk, or even approximate a semi-normal life? This is where the encouragement and input from the medical staff really made a difference for me. They conveyed a feeling of confidence and support that made me want to try even though I did not know how far I would be able to go. Personal relationships were as important emotionally as life supports were physically.

There was a critical turning point in my attitude when I began to attain some degree of independence. I became angry. I could not verbalize this anger, but it was there. It began to consume me. I went through the range of emotions, such as bitterness, hatred, disappointment, and fear. Here I was, 21 years old, a vegetable. How could I go on? I had a choice again: either rise above it or die emotionally, physically, or both. I chose to live, to figuratively reach out and grasp whatever bit of life I could. I attribute this choice primarily to my experience as a member of the track team, where I had to be independent and reach inside to tap resources I did not think were there, to go the extra mile.

However, having made the choice, I still had to have the external motivation to go on. My nurses provided that. They were realistic, nonpatronizing, attentive, and made me work hard. I saw them in the same light as a coach who was there to help me win. At the same time, they gave me constant input. Again, being unable to verbalize, I was in need of monitoring from the outside world. It is terrifying to think what would have happened to me if I was ignored.

I often wonder how many severely injured or ill people live in isolation and become stagnant because they are nonresponsive like I was. This is the thought I carry with me to this day: how lucky I was that people did care. During my hospitalization, my fraternity brothers maintained a constant vigil. Their presence was an additional support to the family and medical personnel, especially during the difficult times when I was faced with major questions, such as, why try or why struggle?

As time passed, my attitudes of hopelessness, hatred, anger, and self-pity began to give way to hope and optimism. In retrospect I believe this can be attributed to the small gains that I was able to make. I could feel and begin to speak, and I regained a variety of body controls. While great gains were not made, there was some significant progress — I began appreciating the fact that I was moving, no matter how slowly.

A traumatizing thought was how I would have coped if I would have had to remain a semi-conscious vegetable for the rest of my life. When I considered the potential realities of what could have happened, I suddenly become most appreciative.

As I reflect upon where I have been and where I am today — able to walk, talk with a slight impediment, and remember most things — I find myself aspiring to qualitative improvements in my life. Although I wish that my speech could continue to improve and that I could walk better, if I had my choice, I would choose speaking clearer over walking better.

Interpersonally, I have many friends, but I am missing one important dimension and that is a girlfriend. Prior to the accident, I had a girlfriend. After it, I did not. At this time, I am my major stumbling block. I cannot see what any girl would see in me. Deep down I guess I am hoping that I will make more gains prior to seeking out a relationship. My rationale is that the more improved I am, the better chance I have of not being rejected. However, I am aware enough to realize that the gains I make may not be tremendous and that I have to accept myself the way I am before another person could accept me. What I have going for me is my ability to place myself in situations where I can learn and experience new things. This is part of my personal rehabilitation effort to maximize my chances for success. I do not know how far I can go but I know that I will try.

Mother's perspective

My son has asked me to record some of my reactions to his accident, illness, hospitalization, and handicap. I look back over the past 2 1/2 years and I find my memory is fragmentary, surrealistic, and shrouded in fog. Therefore,

I will present these thoughts as chronologically as I can, but in a more or less stream-of-consciousness style; that is the way I remember them.

The call from the accident room of the medical center came at 6:40 p.m. on a Tuesday. The doctors reported that our son's condition was grave and that he had stopped breathing several times. I felt very calm as I reminded the doctor that he had been an associate of my late father and that I wished everything possible to be done for my son. My husband and I rushed to the hospital praying and fearful.

Our son was in the critical care section, convulsing and surrounded by aides, doctors, nurses, tubes, machines, and wires. His father was sure he would live; I was sure he would die.

The rest of the night was unreal: we learned as much as we could about the accident, we called our daughter, relatives, and physicians, we signed papers, and we listened to reports of a 5% chance to live.

The worst was that there was nothing I could do but wait helplessly. During the month while he was in a coma, I waited. Through several infections, operations, X-rays, I waited. I asked, "Why?" There was no answer. I was terrified and still there was so very little I could actively do.

School began and I returned to work. This was a great help to me; my mind was occupied and I was active. We all experienced a sort of yo-yo condition: up with hope one day, down with despair the next.

Friends, students, acquaintances, and relatives were extremely supportive. Finally, Ted came to. His eyes opened and he moved — not much, but a little. He would blink twice for "no" and once for "yes." I had hoped it would be like a soap opera where he would open his eyes, say, "Where am I?" and get up out of bed and come home. If I had only known how very long it would be! He was moved from CCU to the neurological section of the hospital. This was somewhat traumatic for us all because the care was not as careful or intensive. At this point, I really came to grips with the problem. I had stopped my why's and self-pity, swallowed some of my overwhelming pride, and accepted the fact that whatever happened, God's will, not mine, would prevail. At last I could cope.

Ted still could not speak, but we discovered he could read. Physical therapy was started; he could sit up with help. He looked awful: retarded and painfully thin. Our physicians were optimistic and had stopped repeating the words, "Condition is stable; he's holding his own; his vital signs are good." How I hated those words! Tubes were removed one at a time; real food was given. I was amused; Ted ate everything. He'd always been an exceedingly fussy eater, and I used to threaten, "Someday you'll be so hungry, you'll eat that!"

On Thanksgiving Day, he came home to dinner. He still could not speak, he had to be tied into the wheelchair so he wouldn't fall out, he had to have a suprapubic catheter, and he had to be fed. But he could smile, he could communicate (sort of), and oh, how he could eat!

From that point on, he came home each Sunday, and by Christmas he could talk — not always intelligibly — but it was still talk. Astonishing to us all was Ted's personality change. He was cheerful, cooperative, and happy (this was very different from the sometimes surly, self-conscious, and somewhat withdrawn person we were used to). Somewhere along the line he'd learned to laugh at himself and to know he had to accept our help.

In February, Ted was allowed to come home for a week. I was very apprehensive about this. He was pretty helpless; he still had a catheter, he was not very mobile, and he had to be dressed. The one thing I'd never wanted to be was a nurse. I always resented sick people and mechanically (with tubes and such) was a klutz. However, I buoyed my sagging confidence by figuring I was as smart as some of the aides who'd been caring for him at the hospital, and we both survived the experience.

It was very difficult to return him to the hospital, but in another month he was home for good. We tried to keep everything as normal as possible. The only physical changes in the house were removing thresholds and one rug and rearranging furniture for easier passage of the wheelchair.

Again, fortune smiled and sent us a young man who stayed with Ted two days a week, a girl one day, and our housekeeper the other two. These individuals were all involved in the rehabilitation process and were inventive therapists. Regardless, I worried and tried to stave off any pitfalls (I am still too protective). Hospital therapy was continued on an outpatient basis, and Ted worked very hard to recover. We all did.

Ted had been at the Medical Center Hospital for 7 months. He received excellent care, and we were supported by the interest and involvement of the entire staff. Everyone, from the lady who pushed the dinner cart to the senior physicians, was exceedingly cooperative. I especially liked the honesty, humor, and realistic approach everyone seemed to have. Questions were always answered. My only problem was in knowing which questions to ask. Our daughter took over at this point. She was preparing for two degrees, one in psychology and one in nursing. She knew what to ask. Her sense of humour also smoothed some rough seas. When her brother started to talk, she spent the afternoon telling him jokes about people with speech impediments. He loved it! Whenever there was a new problem, his sister found the books that would help us study and learn.

Ted's physical progress was coming along. I hoped to keep his mind active and I pushed him to plan to return to school. I shuddered when he could not do things which seem so easy to those who have no physical handicaps, but I tried to be less fearful for him. We took him to restaurants, stores, and sports events so that he'd be used to society. He moved from the wheelchair to crutches and eventually he participated as an attendant in a friend's wedding. Everyone was ecstatic.

Ted returned to college, commuting for the first semester and living at his fraternity the second. He graduated; out of 1600 black-clad seniors, he was the one with a crutch.

Now he walked, talked understandably, had a part-time job, and was accepted to graduate school. It was difficult for me to let him go to an unfamiliar big city with so many problems, but I felt that he had to be independent and live his own life. He does.

How do I feel now? I have intense pride in his achievements and his hard work. I am greatly indebted to so many people for their interest and support. Most of all I'm grateful he has been able to recover and that his family, my husband, daughter, and I, have had the resources to help him. I hurt when he falls, but I try to accept it. We all try to be as realistic as possible about the future and to face it all with gratitude, faith, and humor. When people ask me how does one survive a period such as this, I quote Pearl Buck, who had one of her suffering characters reply, "I really cannot face it, but I must."

Father's perspective

I was working in the garden when my wife came running out screaming, "Teddy's had a motorcycle accident and it's bad." I went cold and thought, "Oh, my God, he's dead. Can Charlotte stand it?"

From then on I did what had to be done, driving cautiously to the emergency room, going to critical care, seeing Teddy, unmarked but mechanized and with blood on his face. I don't remember my thoughts. I do recall thinking, he's not dead yet. I called people including my sister-in-law, but I don't remember what I said. Teddy's sister and her friends arrived. We sat in the CCU waiting room with the others. It was a close community; we became closer.

There were the crises. I prayed he would die rather than become a vegetable. I don't remember the point at which I knew he would not die. It wasn't many days after the accident. At that time, I came back to reality and realized what was and what might be. I cried.

From then on life was a treadmill on which I thought of the outcome as little as possible. The details of the first 6 months or so are blurred. I probably prefer it that way.

As Teddy improved, my biggest concern was how much his intellectual and reasoning faculties were damaged? And if they were not, what dents would being crippled put in his psyche?

My background as an engineer put a lot of trust in absolutes — if this is done, that will result. Although I know what statistics are, the 2-year limit on improvement weighed heavily. Would he improve to the point where he would see the future as promising?

At the present stage in his recovery, I'm sure he has answered the questions I had, and if no further physical improvement is made, he'll still be able to make his way. The fact that I see continuing improvement is just added frosting on a cake that is already much larger than I dared hope.

Discussion questions on the personal statement

1. How would your family respond if you were head-injured while riding a motorcycle after they told you never to ride one?

2. What are the assets and liabilities of being strong-willed and determined not to be a vegetable?
3. How did Ted's parent's personalities and resources complement each other?
4. Why was the family able to respond in a unified manner?
5. How do you think they would have responded if Ted did not make the great gains that he did?
6. How could an engineering perspective as presented by Ted's father be helpful or frustrating in coping with the complexities of brain injury or any other disability?
7. Compare your family's coping style, life values, and resources to Ted's?
8. How would your family respond in this situation?
9. What would they need to cope and maintain their quality of life?
10. How do you think this family would respond if the mother, father, or sister became disabled of if they became brain injured?

Set 7. Prime of life

Perspective

Brain injury never occurs at a convenient time in a person's life. Having read the prior personal statement, try to imagine what your life would have been like if you experienced an injury when you were a young adult.

Exploration

1. If you were as severely injured would your girlfriend or boyfriend remain with you?
2. Would you prefer to be at home or away from home during your rehabilitation?
3. Would your family have responded in a similar or dissimilar manner?
4. What would you have needed to maintain a sense of control, independence, and dignity?
5. Should people who do not wear helmets when riding a motorcycle be covered by insurance or be eligible to sue if injured?
6. How would you respond if your son was brain injured as a result of a motorcycle accident, made great gains, and then wanted to buy another motorcycle so he could feel normal again?
7. What is the responsibility and liability of a person who gives a ride to someone and he or she is brain injured?
8. Do parents have the right to request that a severely brain-injured child not be resuscitated or brought to a hospital? If such a request is made and the child is given medical care over the objections of the parents, who should be responsible for the lifelong care of the child?

References

Allen, K., Linn, R., Gutierrez, H., and Willer, (1994) Family burden following traumatic brain injury, *Rehabil. Psychol.*, 39, 29–48.

Armstrong, C. (1991) Emotional changes following brain injury: psychological and neurological components of depression, denial, and anxiety, *J. of Rehabil.*, April/May/June, 15–21.

Bray, G.P. (1977) Reactive patterns in families of the severely disabled, *Rehabil. Counseling Bull.*, March, 236–239.

Caplan, E. (1976) The family as a support system, in *Support Systems and Mutual Help*, Caplan, E. and Killilea, M., Eds., Grune and Stratton, New York, 19–36.

Carter, R.T. and Cook, R.T. (1991) A culturally relevant perspective for understanding the career paths of visible racial/ethnic group people, in *Adult Career Development*, Leibowitz, Z. and Lea, D., Eds., National Career Development Association, submitted.

Cavallo, M. and Savcedo, C. (1995) Traumatic brain injury in families from culturally diverse populations, *J. of Head Trauma Rehabil.*, 10, 66–77.

Cavallo, M.M., Kay, T., and Ezrachi, O. (1992) Problems and changes after traumatic brain injury: Differing perceptions within and between families, *Brain Injury*, 6(4), 327–335.

Christopherson, V. (1962) The patient and family, *Rehabil. Lit.*, February, 34–41.

Chwallisz, K. (1992) Perceived stress and caregiver burden after brain injury: a theoretical integration, *Rehabil. Psychol.*, 37, 189–201.

Dillard, J.M. (1983). *Multi-Cultural Counseling*, Nelson Hall, Chicago.

Epperson, M. (1977) Families in sudden crisis, *Soc. Work in Health Care*, 2–3, 265–273.

Giacquinta, B. (1977) Helping families face the crisis of cancer, *Am. J. of Nursing*, October, 1585–1588.

Howell, C. (1978) Brain damage, in *Disability and Rehabilitation Handbook*, Godenson, R.M., Ed., McGraw-Hill, New York, 284–295.

Jacobs, H., Muir, C., and Cline, J. (1986) Family reactions to persistent vegetative state, *J. of Head Trauma Rehabil.*, 1(1), 55–62.

Keydel, C.F. (1991) An exploration of perception and coping behavior in family members living with a closed head injured relative, unpublished.

Kosciulek, J. (1994) Relationship of family coping with head injury to family adaptation, *Rehabil. Psychol.*, 39, 215–230.

Kreuter, M., Sullivan, M., Dahllof, A., and Siosteen, A. (1998) Partner relationships, functioning, mood and global quality of life in persons with spinal cord injury and traumatic brain injury, *Spinal Cord*, 36, 252–261.

Kreutzer, J., Devany, C., and Bergquist, S. (1994) Family needs following brain injury: a quantitative analysis, *J. of Head Trauma Rehabil.*, 9, 104–115.

Lezak, M. D. (1986), Psychological implications of traumatic brain damage for the patient's family, *Rehabil. Psychol.*, 31(4), 241–250.

MacFarlene, M. (1999) Treating brain-injured clients and their families, *Fam. Ther.*, 26, 13–30.

Mathis, M. (1984) Personal needs of family members of critically ill patients with and without acute brain injury, *J. of Neurosurg. Nursing*, 16, 36–44.

McKinlay, W. and Hickox, A. (1988) How can families help in the rehabilitation of the head injured?, *J. of Head Trauma Rehabil.*, 3(4), 64–72.

Mitiguy, J.S. (1990) Coping with survival, *Headlines*, 228.

Orsillo, S.M., McCaffrey, R.J., and Fisher, J.M. (1991) The impact of brain injury on the family, *J. of Brain Injury*, 2(4), 19–24.

Orsillo, S.M., McCaffrey, R.J., and Fisher, J.M. (1993) Siblings of head-injured individuals: a population at risk, *J. of Head Trauma Rehabil.*, 8(1), 102–115.

Pearlin, L.I. and Schooler, C. (1978) The structure of coping, *J. of Health and Hum. Behav.*, 19, 2–21.

Rape, R.N., Bush, J.P., and Slavin, L.A. (1992) Toward a conceptualization of the family's adaptation to a member's brain injury: a critique of developmental stage models, *Rehabil. Psychol.*, 37(1), 3–22.

Rocchio, C. (1998) Can families manage behavioral programs in home settings, *Brain Injury Source*, Brain Injury Association, 2(4), 34–35.

Rolland, J. (1994) *Families, Illness and Disability*, Basic Books, New York.

Romano, M. (1974) Family response to traumatic brain injury, *Scandinavian J. of Rehabil. Med.*, (6), 1–4.

Rosenthal, M. and Young, T. (1988) Effective family intervention after traumatic brain injury: theory and practice, *J. of Head Trauma Rehabil.*, 3(4), 41–50.

Waaland, P.K. and Kreutzer, J.S. (1988) Family response to childhood traumatic brain injury, *J. of Head Trauma Rehabil.*, 3(4), 51–63.

Williams, J.M. and Kay, T. (1991) *Brain Injury: A Family Matter*, Paul H. Brookes Publishing Company, Baltimore.

Zarski, J., DePompai, R., and Zook, A. (1988) Traumatic brain injury: dimensions of family responsivity, *J. of Head Trauma Rehabil.*, 3(4), 31–41.

Zeigler, E.A. (1987) Spouses of persons who are brain injured: overlooked victims, *J. of Rehabil.*, 53, 50–53.

part two

Interventions

chapter five

Family assessment

The family is assuming a greater role in the treatment, adjustment, and rehabilitation of people with brain injuries. Increased attention is now given to families in order to assist family members in learning how to adapt to and manage the disabilities within the family systems (Brooks et al., 1987; DeJong et al., 1990; Durgin, 1989; Jacobs, 1984; Livingston and Brooks, 1988; McKinlay and Hickox, 1988; Quine, Pierce, and Lyle, 1988; Sachs, 1985; Schwentor and Brown, 1989).

For those families who are involved in the life care management of a family member with a brain injury, a family assessment is often a key ingredient in developing an effective intervention and management plan (Koch et al., 1995). Family assessment should be an ongoing process because of the episodic nature of the effects of a brain injury, which may result in shifting family roles and the sudden emergence of crisis situations (Sander and Kreutzer, 1999). Therefore, it is important to understand the extent to which the family can support and follow through with specific management interventions in the home (Schwentor and Brown, 1989). A family assessment can also identify current functioning, the family members' expectations for recovery, and their needs for services. In other words, an assessment with the family is an information-obtaining approach that establishes the foundation for appropriate intervention (Kreutzer et al., 1987; Kreutzer et al., 1988; Sherer et al., 1998).

There are many ways to conduct a family assessment. Some include standardized and quantifiable methods such as a self-report, which employs questionnaires that ask for an individual's perception of the family's functioning (Bishop and Miller, 1988; Urbach et al., 1994). Another approach is an observation where the family is observed in the home carrying out assigned tasks designed specifically for them. Another family assessment method is interviewing the family in the home setting. An assessment conducted in the home enables the interviewer to evaluate areas such as individual dynamics, family interaction, living arrangements, environment, and resources. With everyone assembled in the home, communication can be encouraged among family members, and the nature of problems arising from the brain injury can be discussed openly. In their own environment, family members are usually more open to the interviewer, more prone to discuss their disability-related problems, and more ready to share information. If possible, all family members who are living in the home or who have almost immediate availability to the family home, should be included when the interview is conducted. At the beginning of any family assessment, the interviewer may be unaware of those persons who have a decided influence on the management of the person with a brain injury. Someone who is missing from the assessment interview could be that person who has a dominating influence on the injured or the family process and who could influence treatment and rehabilitation outcomes.

While doing a family assessment, it is helpful for the interviewer to follow structured guidelines. In an article focusing on the assessment of families with a brain-injured member, Schwentor and Brown (1989) stress the need for "multiple methods, tools and sources of information" (p. 13).

An assessment approach

In order to be effective and relevant while working with the family coping with a brain injury, the health and human care professional should understand the dynamics that are unique to each family. The following general assessment approach explores this information and focuses on the unique characteristics of the family. It can identify those areas of family life that may be negatively influencing the patient's adjustment, and, in turn, indicate those factors in the family constellation that could promote the adaptation of family members.

The following information represents suggested family assessment guidelines which can serve as an outline when taking a family history.

I. Family Demographic Information and Other Considerations
   A. Ages and genders of family members
   B. Occupations of spouses and family
   C. Educational backgrounds of parents and siblings
   D. Ethnicity
   E. Religion
   F. How many family members contribute to the family income?
   G. How long has the family lived in its present location?
   H. Are relatives living nearby and available in time of crisis?
   I. Who pays the bills in the family?
   J. Does the family have adequate medical insurance coverage?
   K. What are the family plans for the future concerning:
      1. Education
      2. Vacation
      3. Retirement
   L. What are the current and future major expenses of the family?
   M. Any prior experience with brain injury?

N. What is the primary role of the person with a brain injury in the family group? For example, is this person left out from family planning?

O. Are there other serious family problems (e.g., alcoholism, drug abuse, mental illness, or other stressors)? How are they connected with the patient's medical or rehabilitation problems?

P. Who is working? What are work hours? How much work-related stress exists?

II. Communication Patterns in the Family
   A. Is there open hostility among family members?
   B. Do the family members appear to provide emotional support for each other? How is this support given?
   C. What activities do family members share together?
   D. Who dominates the family discussions? Who most frequently contradicts the dominant influence?
   E. Do all family members express their opinions readily or is someone the spokesperson for the family?
   F. Do individual schedules permit much time together at home as a family?
   G. What are the communication of feelings toward the person coping with brain injury?
   H. How would one describe the sibling relationship?
   I. Are there any current areas of family satisfaction?
   J. Is there any communication with extended family?

III. Division of Labor in the Family
   A. What were the roles of parents and children in the family before brain injury? What is to be done, who is to do it, and who takes leadership in deciding on allocation of tasks?
   B. What kinds of things are people expected to do around the house?
   C. Which family members work together?
   D. As a result of the brain injury, have family roles remained flexible or rigid? What role shifts have occurred?
   E. Who is responsible for transportation?

IV. Extent of Family Members' Outside Socialization and Access to Social and Cultural Experiences
   A. Quantity
   B. Quality

V. Health or Illness
   A. Do family members have regular clinic or doctor appointments? Adequate medical insurance?
   B. Are there any previous serious illness/disabilities in the family? If so, what are the family members' feelings about their experiences with doctors and hospitals?

C. What are the general attitudes toward pain, loss, disability, treatment plans, or a specific illness? For example, do family members believe that the particular illness is amenable to treatment or that treatment will lead to better health?

VI. Characteristics of the Brain Injury
   A. What are the physical and emotional consequences of brain injury?
   B. What was the age of the person when the brain injury occurred?
   C. How is the person limited emotionally, physically, intellectually, and vocationally?
   D. What was the cause of the brain injury? What were the situation, circumstances, and responsibility?
   E. What information does the family have about the nature and implications of brain injury?
   F. What are the attitudes of significant others toward brain injury?
   G. What are the family members' perceptions of the future limiting aspects of the patient as a result of brain injury?

VII. Impact of Brain Injury on the Family
   A. Impact on the regular performance of duties within the home
   B. Impact on the activities of family members outside of the home
   C. Do the family members identify any continued adjustment problems resulting from the brain injury?
   D. What information does the family have about brain injury?
   E. Has there been a change in living arrangements since the injury for the person with the brain injury?
   F. Has the person with the brain injury become more dependent on the family since the injury?
   G. Overall, what are the most important changes that have occurred in your family since the injury?
   H. What has your family found helpful in adapting?
   I. What impact has your child's injury had on the family life?
   J. Are community agencies used? Do they seem to be adequate?
   K. What are expectations of family members for each other?
      1. Toward household duties
      2. Maintaining social contacts
      3. Vocational goals
   L. How have the family members accepted the financial restrictions, if any, imposed by the brain injury?
   M. What is the perception of family members regarding their resources in dealing with the brain injury?
   N. How does each family member describe how he or she is dealing with the presence of brain injury in the family?
   O. Who do family members believe is the best person to care for the person with a brain injury?
   P. Has there been a realignment of family goals?

Q. Do family members refer to past areas of satisfaction, including previous successful experiences with crises?

R. Is there a great deal of guilt, shame, and feelings of frustration among family members?

VIII. Appraisal of the Residual Health of the Family Relationships
A. What areas of the marital and parental interaction and shared functioning are least damaged?
B. What areas are most damaged?

IX. Appraisal of the Damage of the Relationships Resulting from the Adjustment to Brain Injury
A. Does brain injury threaten to engulf all major aspects of the marital and parental interactions, or are its effects relatively circumscribed?
B. Are there clear signs of a push toward isolation, disintegration, or regression in the family relationships?

Thematic to these different assessment areas are the issues of family communication and expectations, information about the brain injury, the way the family utilizes external resources, family needs related to the brain injury, and the changes that have occurred in the family since the onset of the injury. These issues provide a focus for assessment and can generate information for the development of assessment approaches. Assessment information also assists in the identification of problem areas relevant to the family and overall life adjustment of the person with a brain injury.

Specific to understanding family dynamics concerning the impact of brain injury is the realization that target assessment areas may differ slightly according to family ethnicity. For many ethnic groups disability is a cultural concept, and those issues that may be significant for one ethnic group may not be for another. Some ethnic groups may use extended family as an expected resource in times of crisis or transition while for other cultural groups extended family may simply be unavailable or may not even be asked to provide support. Yet within each ethnic group there are intra-group differences, a diversity determined by cultural history and values, social-political conditions, social environments, and economic conditions. Importantly, acculturation issues that may be integral to family values need to be identified for they may suggest the family's willingness to participate in treatment planning.

Conclusion

All of these identified areas emerging from family assessment may pinpoint both the family strengths and problems that are relevant to appropriate intervention. Building on the family's capabilities to manage the brain trauma situation, and linking these assets to problem solving efforts, may also provide the basis for a suggested intervention approach. Yet in response to many of these assessment areas, family members may have difficulty answering precisely. The interviewer should both ask the family members to elaborate their responses, while at the same time be sensitive to the feelings of family members. The family may be resistant to any intervention efforts, and support and reassurance should be given to help comfort and reinforce the family for their own caregiving efforts. Moreover, special consideration should be given to the presence of other stressors that are not directly related to the brain injury situation (other family health problems, unemployment). It is also important to consider that interviews with extended family members may provide useful intergenerational information in identifying both strengths and weaknesses in the family (Schwentor and Brown, 1989). A major contribution in the area of interviewing is the research on the Head Injury Family Interview (Hi-Fi) developed by The Research and Training Center on Head Trauma and Stroke at the New York University Medical Center (Kay et al., 1993).

There are many challenges in implementing a viable and reasonable treatment-rehabilitation plan for families and persons who are living with the impact of brain injury. A primary step in this process is an assessment approach that is responsive to the many influences that impact the head injured family member, the total family system, and their mutual needs.

The following personal statement, *We're Tough, A Wife's Perspective*, explores the impact of a severe brain injury on familial roles, the ongoing stress related to coping and surviving, and the power of a religious-cultural perspective.

Personal statement
We're tough, a wife's perspective

I am a 45-year-old woman whose husband of 24 years suffered a traumatic brain injury (TBI) 3 years ago. At the time of his injury, we lived in a large house in the suburb of a midwestern city surrounded by other families of the Orthodox Jewish faith. I was preparing for the empty nest and had gone to college to get a degree in interior decoration. Our older daughter was in her senior year in college and our younger daughter was in her senior year in high school. I was going to have a lot of time on my hands with the girls gone and I looked forward to having a career and spending more time with my husband. He was an executive in an accounting firm and he was very busy with work and in our synagogue. Everyone admired and respected him, but he had very little time to spend at home. He had promised to give up some of his religious activities and spend more time with me. Little did I know that soon he would be spending all his time with me and it wouldn't be a happy time!

Our lives changed drastically one night 3 years ago. It was a slippery winter night. I tried to convince my husband to cancel his meeting that night;

he insisted on going but promised to come home early. The next thing I knew I was rushing to our local hospital emergency ward where I was told that he had been in a bad collision, had suffered a severe brain injury and probably wouldn't live. For days he hovered between life and death. The whole Jewish community prayed for him. He was in a coma for 3 weeks, but he lived. When he finally woke up, it was like a miracle, but we weren't prepared for the way he was. He tried to hit the nurses and said things to people that he never would have said before the accident. He was a stranger. My daughters couldn't take it; they didn't want to go to the hospital. After the acute phase, he was in the rehabilitation hospital for 6 months and then finally he came home. I think I neglected my daughters during that time and I feel bad about that. All I could think about was my husband though I know they never got the attention children in their senior years should get. They don't say anything about it, but I think they resent the fact that I wasn't excited about their activities. I couldn't even get involved in my younger daughter's trip to Israel that summer. But what about me? One day I have a husband who is the strength of the family, who makes everyone proud, and the next, I have this person who scares everyone with his temper and who thinks everything is fine when really it's a sorry mess.

Life is getting better. The two of us get along. Sometimes I even like the fact that my husband is around all the time. He can be good company, but he can also be very difficult, almost impossible at times. He has a lot of anger and frustration, but he won't face that yet. He still has trouble controlling his temper; he says whatever he thinks and frequently insults people. His daughters do not like to stay alone with him because he tries to do things that are dangerous like walking outside without his cane. When they try to talk him out of it, he gets furious, says insulting things to them, and does whatever he pleases. He can't face reality yet. He wants to go back to work, but he can't remember things from one minute to the next. He is still very intelligent but in the middle of what you think is a very reasonable comment, he'll say something foolish, but he doesn't realize it. He thinks that he is making good sense. You can't tell him anything in a critical way; he becomes a "crazy man."

We had to move to a one-story house, out of our old neighborhood. That was also very hard on the girls. Fortunately, my husband's business had excellent health insurance so we didn't have to go into debt. They also had a good disability plan which we can live on, but things are still very tight. Everyone says I should get someone to stay with my husband so I can go out, but that's expensive. Besides, I wouldn't trust most people to know how to handle him, especially when he's difficult. The girls think that I should get him to go to a therapist, that he could be helped to control his temper and to remember better. Maybe I will one of these days. Health insurance would help pay for that. I recently joined a support group. It feels like I am associating with a whole new social group, people who are down and out, so to speak. I joined because I hoped that it would be a way to find out about community resources for the head injured. There doesn't seem to be much out there. Some people in the support group trade respite care with each other but I don't think my husband would like spending time with a stranger. They wouldn't have anything in common. I'm particularly worried about the future when I get too old to take care of him. Of course my daughters will always be available, but they'll have their own families and their father would be an extra burden. I would never put him in a home unless I absolutely had to.

I guess we'll be a good old twosome until the day we die. Once in a great while, I do things with my friends and I have my needlework. I'm not unhappy. My ancestors were all tough. Life is hard. I'm a survivor.

Discussion questions on the personal statement

1. Reflecting on the assessment approach discussed in this chapter, what important issues emerge in this personal statement?
2. How does religion impact coping with a brain injury?
3. What are the unique stressors related to the onset of a parental brain injury when a couple has reached the end of the child rearing stage?
4. What did the wife mean by the statement, "He was a stranger?" How does this reality challenge the resources of the non-injured spouse?
5. Discuss the advantages and disadvantages of having a person with a brain injury around all of the time?
6. How can a family protect a person with a brain injury while trying to have the person live as independently as possible?
7. How would this family cope if they did not have excellent health insurance?
8. What are the factors to be considered when developing a long-range plan that meets the needs of the person who has a brain injury as well as the needs of the primary caregiver?
9. How can traditions and cultural expectations be an asset or a liability?

Set 8. Rain or shine

Perspective

One way to gain a perspective on the family challenged by a brain injury is to explore how families function when life is ideal or not so ideal. Often, when families are in a state of crisis they lose contact with their pre-trauma reality and tend to believe that, prior to head trauma, their life was more functional, fulfilling, and rewarding. Conversely, if the trauma did not occur, they believe that their life would be more fulfilling, satisfying, and rewarding.

Exploration

1. List five qualities that define your family.

2. If you have experienced a brain injury, were these qualities altered or changed?
3. What are the abilities needed by a family to negotiate the perils of the brain injury experience?
4. Are the responses to a brain injury different or similar to other traumas and losses?
5. Should divorce be considered as a reasonable alternative for someone married to a person with severe brain injury?
6. Should divorce be considered as a reasonable alternative for someone married to a person who has Alzheimer's Disease, AIDS, or a spinal cord injury?
7. Is the stress experienced by a family challenged by a brain injury different from the stress related to other illnesses or disabilities? If so, in what ways?
8. Identify and discuss other familial factors that can intensify the stress associated with brain injury.
9. Assuming that self-help and informational programs were available and accessible to families challenged by brain injury, do you believe that all families would benefit from these resources?
10. Some families cope with the brain injury experience by wanting, needing, and perusing all relevant information. Other families see information as distressing and overwhelming. Do you feel that information is always helpful to families? If so, why? If not helpful, address.
11. If you were or are brain injured, what are or would be the sick role expectation your family has/would have for you?
12. Should people who are severely brain injured have their sexual needs and issues addressed by family members as well as professionals?
13. How would your family respond if you were hypersexual and at risk to contract AIDS?
14. How would your family respond if you were married to a person with a severe brain injury and you told them you were using alcohol to cope?

Set 9. Good feelings, bad feelings

Perspective

The awareness that families have different attitudes and feelings to each other individually and/or collectively is an important point to consider when addressing the needs of the person with brain injuries as well as the family. For example, all persons with a brain injury do not love their spouses, children, and families. Similarly, not all families love, care about, or want to respond to the needs of a person with a brain injury. The following questions will facilitate discussion of this point and identify many areas that are critical in the assessment process.

Exploration

1. How should a family respond to a mother who abandoned them 20 years earlier and is now seeking a reconciliation since she was in a car accident and had severe brain injury?
2. What would you advise a friend whose brain-injured parent sexually abused him or her as a child and now wants to move in so he or she can be with the grandchildren?
3. What should a woman do to meet the needs of her brain-injured sister who paid her tuition so she could go to medical school? (Her husband dislikes his sister-in-law since her brain injury and said he would leave if his wife gets involved.)
4. What should a child do when his or her mother remarries and after one year her new husband has severe brain injury? This is complicated by the fact that the mother left her first husband because she could not deal with his brain injury. Consequently, the children took care of their father until he committed suicide.
5. Identify and discuss the community resources available in your area that could meet the needs of your family if you experienced a severe brain injury.
6. If you experienced a brain injury today, how would you accept and cope with the losses?
7. Would family responses to your brain injury be different today than 10 years ago? Why?
8. What kind of information related to brain injury would be helpful to you and your family?
9. What kind of information would not be helpful?
10. How would your family respond if you were unable to adjust to your brain injury and you became a source of conflict in the family?
11. In what way does ethnic background impact a family's response to loss or brain injury?
12. What are the problems and needs of a family who must deal with other stressors such as alcoholism while living with a family member who is head injured?
13. What activities can a post-injury family engage in to promote a quality of life?
14. What would a home visit by a health care worker reveal about your family?
15. What are your family's fondest memories?
16. How would a brain injury to a family member alter your family's goals?
17. What emotions would your family have a difficult time sharing?
18. Which family values would you want in your future?
19. Have these or would these values assist you in coping with the demands and losses associated with a brain injury?

20. Who in your family could cope with a major loss with the best attitude? Why?

References

Bishop, D.S. and Miller, I.W. (1988) Traumatic brain injury: empirical family assessment techniques, *J. of Head Trauma Rehabil.*, 3, 4, 16–30.

Brooks, N., Campsie, L., Symington, C., Beattie, A., and McKinlay, W. (1987) The effects of severe brain injury on patient and relative within seven years of injury, *J. of Head Trauma Rehabil.*, 2(3), 1–13.

DeJong, G., Batavia, A.I., and Williams, J.M. (1990) Who is responsible for the lifelong well being of a person with a brain injury?, *J. of Head Trauma Rehabil.*, 5(1), 9–22.

Durgin, C.J. (1989) Techniques for families to increase their involvement in the rehabilitation process, *Cognit. Rehabil.*, May–June, 22–25.

Jacobs, H.E. (1984) The family as a therapeutic agent: long term rehabilitation for traumatic brain injury patients, National Institute of Handicapped Research.

Kay, T., Cavallo, M.M., and Ezrachi, O. (1993) Administration manual, N.Y.U. brain injury family interview, New York University Medical Center, Research and Training Center on Head Trauma and Stroke, New York.

Koch, L., Merz, M., and Lynch, R. (1995) Screening for mild traumatic brain injury: a guide for rehabilitation counselor, *J. of Rehabil.*, 61, 50–56.

Kreutzer, J., Leininger, B., Doherty, K., and Waaland, P. (1987) General health and history questionnaire, Medical College of Virginia, Rehabilitation Research and Training Center on Severe Traumatic Brain Injury, Richmond, VA.

Kreutzer, J., Camplair, P., and Waaland, P. (1988) Family needs questionnaire, Medical College of Virginia, Rehabilitation Research and Training Center on Severe Traumatic Brain Injury, Richmond, VA.

Livingston, M.G. and Brooks, D.N. (1988) The burden on families of the brain injured: a review, *J. of Head Trauma Rehabil.*, 3(4), 6–15.

McKinlay, W. and Hickox, A. (1988) How can families help in the rehabilitation of the head injured?, *J. of Head Trauma Rehabil.*, 3(4), 64–72.

Quine, S., Pierce, J.P., and Lyle, D.M. (1988) Relatives as lay-therapists for the severely head-injured, *Brain Injury*, 2, 139–149.

Sachs, P.R. (1985) Beyond support: traumatic brain injury as a growth experience for families, *Rehabil. Nursing*, 10(1), 21–23.

Sander, A. and Kreutzer, J. (1999) A holistic approach to family assessment after brain injury, in *Rehabilitation of the Adult and Child with Traumatic Brain Injury*, 3rd ed., Rosenthal, M., Griffith, E., Kreutzer, J., and Pentland, B., Eds., F.A. Davis, Philadelphia.

Schwentor, D. and Brown, P. (1989) Assessment of families with a traumatically brain-injured relative, *Cognit. Rehabil.*, 8–14.

Sherer, M., Oden, K., Bergloff, P., Levin, E., and High, W. (1998) Assessment and treatment of imposed awareness after brain injury: implications for community re-intergration, *Neuro Rehabil.*, 10, 25–38.

Urbach, J., Sonenklar, N., and Culbert, J. (1994) Risk-factors and assessment in children of brain-injured parents, *J. of Neuropsychiart.*, 6, 289–295.

chapter six

Brain injury and family intervention

Many specific interventions for the person with a brain injury have recently been identified (Hart and Jacobs, 1993; Marmé and Skord, 1993; Medlar, 1993; Bullook et al., 1998). This awareness supports the belief that families play a significant role in both the present and future life of the person with brain injury. Families find themselves providing perpetual care and treatment to a "transformed" family member. For family members the behavioral, emotional, and cognitive problems are usually the most difficult to manage, and the hidden financial, physical, and emotional costs associated with caring for a brain-injured survivor often impair or even destroy the family unit (Jacobs, 1984). Helping a family adjust to the impact of a brain injury requires an appropriate course of action, and through this intervention caregivers can be helped to function more effectively and efficiently in their demanding and changing roles.

The struggle by family members to achieve adaptive roles involves an ongoing process of dealing with the many problems that result from living with a person with brain injury. These problems include the possible social isolation of family members, the constant demand to carry out the prescribed treatment regimen, managing the family member's own grief, dealing with unpredictable behavior, and assuming the burden of caregiving responsibilities (Zeigler, 1989; Dombouy et al., 1997). The continued inclination to become overinvolved with the person with brain injury and the ever-present reality that the person with brain injury might draw attention away from other marital and family needs should be considered.

Chapters six and seven explore different intervention strategies. The two chapters focus on alleviating problems and optimizing opportunities generated by living with a person with a brain injury. The overall goal is to support the family, as well as help family members minimize their own disability-related problems. Chapter six identifies theoretical assumptions for intervention, particular intervention goals for families attempting to adjust to the brain injury trauma, and specific tasks to accomplish these goals. Chapter

seven presents group counseling as a key component of treatment and rehabilitation. These intervention considerations which apply to most families
as they live with the person who is gradually meeting treatment and rehabilitation objectives, include specific situations that necessitate a particular
helping approach. These situations, which arise from living the brain injury
experience, are unexpected family crises and stress of coping with the reality
of permanent loss. Both of these realities call for special skills when developing a helping approach.

Theoretical assumptions

For an intervention approach to be effective, certain assumptions are critical
to an intervention with families of persons with a brain injury.

1. An intervention effort directed toward the person and family is a joint
   venture shared by the health care and rehabilitation professional and
   the family members. If the person, family members, and professional
   worker share their energy and resources, it will facilitate the attainment of common goals. It is important to emphasize that the family
   is an integral part of the helping process, and most individuals cannot
   be treated in isolation even if they are severely limited by a brain
   injury. If they become partners in intervention, stabilization, and rehabilitation efforts, the family members generally develop more willingness to work with each other. This is particularly true when family
   members choose between competing goals and values as they attempt
   to cope with the reality of brain injury. The degree of consensus that
   develops among family members regarding the ranking of family
   goals can be a crucial factor in the family's ability to deal successfully
   with adjustment demands. What often fosters this consensus is the
   mutuality that has already been established between the health care
   worker and the family (Pieper and Singer, 1991).
2. There will be predictable points of family stress when coping with
   brain injury. Each of these points must be examined individually
   because each can bring unique problems. For example, discharge
   planning can surface many unresolved issues regarding family roles
   during the rehabilitation process. Also, additional problems can be
   created when the person with a brain injury is at home because caring
   responsibilities may force family members to assume different functions in the home (MacFarlene, 1999).
3. The basic instinct of people under stress is to hold to previously
   proven patterns of action, whether they are effective or not. A family
   reactive pattern usually will not vary from the past. Health care professionals should make an effort during family assessment to understand these past adjustment styles and be aware of how they influence
   the present (Coppa et al., 1999).

4. Rehabilitation is generally a process of teaching persons how to manage their disabilities in their own environments. The key to coping with one's disability is to receive enough satisfactions and rewards to make life worthwhile (Treischmann, 1974; Pieper, 1991). When reinforcements for the person are withdrawn from the family environment, he or she may feel isolated and become reluctant to respond to treatment efforts, or may become more manipulative in attempts to gain attention. The complexity of brain injury is that the family must accept and process the loss of the preinjury person and accept the new person in the family. For some family systems this is a manageable task; for others it is an illusive dream or an unending nightmare.

5. Intervention programs that aim to increase caregiver's knowledge and/or perceived social support can consist of presentations, discussion groups, and support groups. A multi-dimensional approach that emphasizes the acquisition of caregiver skills through periodic interaction with those who have experience in dealing with brain injury within the family can assist family members to manage the different problems resulting from the disability. Further, those caregivers who have been socialized to be more passive and accepting of things as they are, may benefit from a support group that provides role models as well as skills related to living in spite of stress, loss, and trauma (Appendices A and B).

Emerging from these assumptions are specific goals for family intervention. Family adaptation to brain injury is ongoing and will stimulate varied family reactions and different adjustment demands. During the unfolding process of family adjustment, there are certain adaptive goals which are ever-present and provoke definite tasks for goal achievement by family members. They are detailed in the following sections.

Providing the family with a sense of competence

The occurrence of a brain injury will increase anxiety for family members and reinforce feelings of sadness, guilt, confusion, isolation, anger, and helplessness. An intervention approach should aid family members to alleviate these feelings and assist them in regaining or developing control of their lives, individually and collectively. The development of such competence usually represents the creation of new, positive family influences on the individual with a brain injury.

The tasks to achieve these competencies include:

1. Learning about the effects of a brain injury and the implications for physical, emotional, and intellectual functioning
2. Learning how to deal with varied management problems accruing from the brain injury

3. Learning different coping strategies that assist family members to handle more effectively daily living concerns
4. Learning how to interact effectively with health professionals and/or members of the rehabilitation team
5. Learning problemsolving skills
6. Learning, when necessary, how to make necessary shifts in role responsibilities

Assisting the family to normalize relations with each other and, as much as possible, with the family member experiencing a brain injury

Normalization is an effort to provide appropriate patterns of expectations from family members for continued activities and maintenance of customary role responsibilities. Normalization does not eliminate the possibility, however, that many families will have to become reoriented to the realities of the brain injury. For family members the problem is usually not brain injury as an abstract concept, but coping with it in every critical aspect of their lives. The tasks that assist family members to achieve normalization include:

1. Give responsibility, when appropriate, to the person for appropriate home duties and a voice in family matters.
2. Understand their own grief reactions and know that such feelings as fear of the future, anger, frustration, and disappointment are to be expected among family members.
3. Understand their own perceptions of what the brain injury means to family life and discuss these perceptions, when appropriate, with other family members.
4. Balance the needs of the person with a brain injury with the needs of other family members.
5. Learn to take care of themselves, their significant others, and their marriage.

Developing a renewed awareness by family members of their own resources and strengths

In their attempts to manage the effects of the brain injury on family life, family members often overlook their own assets and strengths in dealing with recurrent problems. The stress induced from living with a person with a brain injury frequently stimulates a continued state of anxiety, which, in turn, clouds the identification of those capabilities which can lead to this awareness. Tasks that can assist family members to attain this goal include an understanding of how past family crises were handled and a recognition of transgenerational coping strategies.

1. Utilize community resources, especially participation in support groups, which can provide feedback to family members on their own capabilities.
2. Enhance their own expectations for each other regarding family tasks and management responsibilities for brain injury.
3. Communicate with each other about their own needs and concerns in living with brain injury.

Creating a consistent, supportive, emotional experience for the family in which their mutual needs and feelings are recognized and acknowledged

Frequently the multi-dimensionality of losses experienced by the person with a brain injury (e.g., those caused by physical restrictions or loss of job due to brain injury) are overlooked by other family members. The person with a brain injury may be hesitant to talk about personal losses because he perceives that other family members will not understand, or will be overwhelmed. Instead, these feelings are suppressed or the person reacts to this family unresponsiveness by exaggerated dependency or continual irritation with others. To create this supportive experience for the family the following tasks can be considered:

1. Learn how to talk with each other about concerns and needs, and provide an atmosphere for this discussion where these feelings, concerns, and needs will not be negatively evaluated.
2. Foster the awareness of mutual respect and recognition of each family member's self-worth.

The focus for all of these identified tasks is on the emerging needs of the family. If the family is to be an important resource in the treatment and/or rehabilitation of the brain-injured family member, then family members will have to acquire certain skills. Each task implies the utilization of an accompanying skill, and apart from the imparting of necessary information to family members about brain injury, much of the intervention efforts will deal with assisting family members to acquire these skills. What skills families need will depend on what has been learned from the family assessment. How emotional problems relevant to the living with the effects of the brain injury are resolved depends on the nature of the problem and its relationship to the trauma. Brain injury alters the family structure, and, consequently, communication patterns can change.

An important issue when considering intervention approaches is the need to be aware of a multicultural perspective when interacting with a family that represents an ethnic minority. There may be language and value differences between the health professionals and family members. The meaning of the cognitive and behavioral disabilities associated with brain injury may reflect the family's combined historical and current experiences. There are also acculturation and racial identity factors that impact on the family's adjustment. It is important for the health professional, consequently, to understand how family members perceive the disability and its implications for family life. This knowledge can then provide a context for planning intervention efforts (Rosenthal et al., 1996).

Intervention can be conducted by rehabilitation and health care professionals or by non-professionals — peers and family. Intervention often begins when a member of the patient's rehabilitation team contacts a professional for possible family assistance. Frequently the rehabilitation team encourages family members to seek short-term assistance in order to deal with both expected and unexpected problems. The family visits may take place in either an office or home setting, and if initiated soon after the onset of brain injury, they should take place as often as possible in order to alleviate family concerns. Intervention usually takes place in a support group setting, and the rehabilitation team may recommend such an opportunity as the individual is undergoing in-patient treatment and family concerns are emerging. Family members may not seek a support group until they are confronted with serious family problems and realize that input from others and the ventilation of their feelings will assist in their own adjustment efforts.

Frequently, families face adjustment difficulties that are perceived to be beyond their internal and external resources. Customary coping styles utilized in the past do not seem to be working to manage serious problems associated with brain injury. A critical situation occurs within the family, and the situation may be viewed as a crisis when increased tension and perhaps family disorganization surrounding adjustment to the brain injury escalate beyond the member's coping ability. The crisis event is not a simple occurence. It is a complex and difficult reality but a situation which may contain either the seeds of family growth and positive change or the stimulus for a complete family breakdown. For the family to adjust successfully to the brain injury trauma, the crisis must be contained.

With a focus on the family's acquisition of adaptive skills to manage a crisis or other trauma-related difficulties, there are three approaches that can be beneficial for helping families both to learn and implement those skills. These three approaches are counseling, education, and support, and they will depend both on what is learned about family needs during the assessment process and the availability of internal and external resources.

Counseling

This intervention is usually oriented to current family functioning, and involves such approaches as providing family members with the opportunity to share their feelings with each other, learning important information about the brain injury process, asking for clarification of issues, and encouraging questions that lead to an understanding of how family members perceive the injury affecting family life and their own expectations. One of the initial goals of counseling, before formal education approaches or formal supports are suggested, is to assist the family members to have trust in the health or human care provider. Another goal is to assist the family members in understanding their own perception of their ability and willingness to provide care for the person with the brain injury and to take care of themselves during the treatment and/or rehabilitation process. Because of the importance for the achievement of these goals, the provider should begin a counseling intervention with the family as soon as possible after the onset of the brain injury. While the individual is undergoing critical care management in the hospital, family members usually need to have questions answered, be reassured, and be told that someone is available to act as a resource for their own emerging problems. This is a very vulnerable time for the family and it has long-term implications and requires immediate intervention. In counseling family members, attempts are made to maintain a listening, non-evaluative posture that encourages the expression of feelings and questions by the family. The service provider needs to develop trust with the family, and often this can be generated by the professional's acceptance of family feelings and illustration of a genuine interest in assisting family members. Counseling also includes helping families to recognize their own strengths, appreciate limitations, and anticipate specific problem areas. Sharing information about the brain injury, as well as varied management issues, helps prepare the family for possible events related to the brain injury that eventually may be of concern to the family.

A helping approach

When a state of crisis is perceived by both the helping professional and family members, there are specific counseling strategies that need to be utilized. Crisis intervention with the family because of brain injury trauma can occur in three phases: the beginning phase, when there is the initial awareness of the trauma; the middle phase, when family members are becoming gradually or suddenly aware of the impact of the trauma on both the patient and family life; and the termination phase, when family members are energetically attempting to steady the chaos caused by the crisis. Each of these phases is relevant to varied forms of family crisis induced by the brain injury. If the family's vulnerable state of equilibrium, for example, is upset by emotional outbursts, dashed expectations, or a sudden financial emergency, then there will be an initial reaction. What follows is a period when family members are aware of the impact of the crisis, and then a time when the crisis is at least temporarily resolved. Each phase, moreover, varies in length, though frequently the crisis of brain injury is long term, thus creating a situation of chronic crisis and long-term need.

Beginning phase

At this time, the family needs primarily the emotional support to focus on the present and to begin to understand their own perceptions of the meaning of what has happened. Before family members can begin to attend to the present and express their own beliefs about what they perceive is the "crisis" for the family, they need someone to simply be with them to attend, listen, and respond to their feelings. Gradually, the family members will want to talk about how this crisis has affected them and the patient, but they first must be convinced that the health professional wishes to listen and share their grief, hope, anger, and disappointment. Listening and acknowledging the legitimacy of family feelings can communicate confidence to the family, and on their part, trust in the helping professional. During their initial reaction to the crisis, family members usually want to ventilate their feelings and need empathy and understanding.

Middle phase

As the family members gradually gain an understanding of the crisis and face the reality of what has happened, they will begin to ask such questions as, what can we do to help the person with a brain injury and how can we manage this disruption to our family life? Feelings of anger, guilt, self-pity, disappointment, sadness, and loss will still continue, but family members will begin to search for answers and explore what are the best ways to cope with this family trauma. The family's search for answers may demand a specific response, but many questions will have no answer. There may be no discernible reason why the brain injury has occurred, but the reality is that it has occurred and if the family and the patient are to survive the crisis must be addressed.

During this intervention state, the health care professional continues to listen, and encourages the family members to understand not only the possible problem areas for adjustment, but also their own internal and external resources that can be utilized to deal with the crisis. With this encouragement, moreover, the concerned and skilled professional can stimulate the family to enter into a dialogue in which mutual feelings can be recognized and different solutions can be shared to the varied problems emerging from the crisis.

As the family begins to more fully understand the meaning of brain injury to family life, certain tasks related to family reorganization may then be assigned. These duties may involve contacting the extended family, performing more chores in the home, or using designated community supports such as local chapters of the Brain Injury Association as well as other resources (Appendices A and B).

The main goal of this phase is to assist the family in adapting to the reality of the crisis. It involves helping the family move from a state of perceived helplessness, confusion, and disorientation to an emotional level where these feelings are minimized. Such additional feelings as anger, guilt, and blame begin to be controlled, and perhaps hope and optimism can emerge.

Termination phase

When the health care professional realizes that family equilibrium is being restored, adjustment problems are being addressed, and family members are involved in many of the solutions to problems emanating from the crisis, continued contact with the family may well depend on the changing needs related to the brain injury process. Given the frequent long term nature of severe brain injury, and the different crises that can unexpectedly occur, most families need long term support. Thus, continued contact from the health care professional will usually be necessary. The terminating phase is more of a journey than a destination.

When considering such process counseling issues as listening, encouraging the expression of questions and emotions, and identifying central problem areas, counseling must continue during the entire span of intervention. The interventions of support and education imply that the process of counseling is still an ongoing reality with the family members.

Education

As a vitally important intervention approach, education can take a number of forms. For example, many rehabilitation treatment centers and other related agencies have formal education programs for family members. During these programs information about brain injury is imparted, family questions are answered, and management techniques are suggested which can deal with such issues as poor attention span, inappropriate social skills, low frustration tolerance, and disorientation and organizational problems. Different community resources are also identified. Many families can benefit from these programs since they can learn problem-solving skills from personnel who are usually extremely knowledgeable about the implications of brain injury for family life. The role of the service provider is helping the family to utilize formal and informal education opportunities. With the knowledge of what education programs are available, the provider can indicate the advantages to family members from their involvement in these activities.

Frequently, however, the health care provider must assume the role of educator since the family may not have the immediate opportunity to take part in any formal program, or information must be imparted that responds to current problems. This information can include a wide scope of topics such as the availability of community resources, the nature of brain injury and the implications of cognitive, emotional, and behavioral deficits on patient and family functioning, the teaching of effective coping skills, insights into how family expectations may have to change, and ways that family members can take care of themselves and their marriage. Financial and legal information may also be included, as well as how issues of blame and guilt can be managed. Education can further include the identification to the family how previous family generations have handled family crises, and what coping resources can be utilized during the present crisis (see Appendices A, B, and C).

The teaching of coping skills is a particularly valuable contribution which health and human care providers can make to the family's adjustment efforts. Coping comprises efforts to manage stressful demands, regardless of outcome. There are many threats and challenges to family life as the result of the brain injury trauma, and families need to evaluate the range of their own coping resources and alternatives. One particular coping strategy during the family's adjustment to brain injury is reframing, namely, attempting to see the patient's behavior in a different light. A family member, through reframing, gives another meaning to the situation. This meaning can be attained with positive comparisons by recognizing some of the patient's negative behaviors as signs of patient progress or becoming convinced that eventually the burdens accruing from patient management and care will diminish. Reframing involves changing one's attitude, focusing on caregiving strengths, and even creating one's own system of affective rewards. Other coping approaches may include the reliance on religious faith, sharing concerns with others, seeking as much information as possible about the injury and its implications for the future, patient functioning, and undertaking rational problemsolving. This problem solving entails talking out the problem, looking at choices, when these are available, and then developing a plan of action to confront and minimize the problem.

Another aspect of educational intervention is teaching family members how to deal and work with health care and rehabilitation professionals. Because of their own anxiety and unfamiliarity with all the issues of brain injury, family members may tend to be reluctant to ask questions or be more assertive during the interactions with the rehabilitation team. Families can be taught to carefully record the different treatment plans that will be undertaken with the injured family member, ask health professionals to repeat unclear statements, and be assertive in seeking information about certain problems that arise as treatment continues. If the family is to successfully negotiate the problems of living with someone with brain injury, questions arising from adjustment and treatment concerns must be asked. Assertiveness and self-advocacy by family members can stimulate the communication, as well as the mutual awareness process.

Support

There are many operational definitions of support, such as the expression of emotional support (esteem, affection, trust); the communication of appraisal support (affirmation, feedback); giving information (advice, suggestions); and providing instrumental support (money, labor, time) (House, 1981). These support types apply to families experiencing the trauma of brain injury, and such supports can be provided by either an individual worker or family support groups. The latter resource frequently addresses those issues faced by family members who have a desire to speak with someone dealing with their own unique collection of problems. Barker (1988) describes the need for involvement with other spouses:

> The only way you can cope with it is to talk with someone who understands, has experienced the same thing, and knows just what the situation is, so that all you have to do sometimes is just say a few words and the other person knows exactly what you're talking about without going into all the details (p. 36).

In brain injury situations, families with good support systems appear to be more successful in overcoming traumatic situations and maintaining a familial sense of competence (Leathem et al., 1996). Keydel (1991), in studying families living with brain injuries, reported that it was the belief that support was available rather than the use of support that was contributing to the alleviation of family stress. Another influence on the perception of social support is the family's belief about the acceptability of asking for support from others. Getting help from others may be perceived in some families as a testimony to the strength and closeness of the family and friendship network; or, the effects of the brain injury on the family may be so traumatizing that family members, in their low feelings of self-esteem, may believe they are not entitled to support, may not ask for it, or may even refuse it when offered (Keydel, 1991).

The timing of providing support, especially in the forms of giving information or urging family members to become involved in family support groups, needs to be handled carefully. In the early stages of brain injury many family members may still need the protective shield of denial and would consequently find information and support groups quite negative. Family members need to feel comfortable when hearing about problems that might still exist many years down the road (Zeigler, 1989). Intervention approaches that emphasize support should include the needs of family members regarding when the communication of information, or hearing how others have dealt with problems, would be most appropriately received.

Whether support takes the form of feedback, reassurance, or advice, the communication of support is an active process that acknowledges the family's abilities and reinforces those aspects of the family's functioning which appear adaptive and beneficial to the treatment process. Support includes helping family members to understand how they are reacting to the trauma, encouraging the expression of family feelings, and helping family members make active decisions in daily care (Sachs, 1991).

Conclusion

Whether intervention consists primarily of counseling, education, or support, it should enable families to attain and maintain a reasonable quality of life. At the same time as they perform their caregiving roles, the family acts as a resource for the potential rehabilitation, growth, and development of the transformed family member. Intervention should be tailored to the individual needs of families and should focus on aiding family members to bring normalcy back into their lives as they respond to caregiving demands. Efforts to regain the balance in family life requires a sense of competency by family members, a consistent emotional experience for the family, and an awareness of their own strengths, limitations, and resources.

The following personal statement, *One More Burden, A Mother's Perspective* presents the challenges faced by a mother whose dreams were shattered. It reflects the complexity of loss, as well as an emerging optimism for the future based upon a unique perspective formulated in difficult circumstances.

Personal statement

One more burden, a mother's perspective

I am a 51-year-old black woman who lives with my daughter in a small house in a quiet section of a southern city. My husband passed away many years ago. I worked as a kitchen helper for many years, but have been unemployed because of serious illnesses and disabilities. I suffer from asthma and a heart condition and receive Social Security Disability Insurance. I walk with great difficulty and I am not able to go up the stairs in my home. I have two other daughters who live nearby. One has completed the 11th grade and the other has completed 9th. Both are unemployed and receiving Aid to Families with Dependent Children because they have children of their own. Both daughters and their children were living with me until the serious accident of my third daughter.

My daughter, 25, was driving when she was hit from behind by a car that ran a stoplight, and she was thrown into the windshield. She was not wearing her seatbelt at the time of the accident, and she suffered a serious brain injury. She spent many months in the hospital. When they discharged her, she came to live with me, and my two daughters had to move out. Since she has been at home, she has been unemployed and has received medical certification that she is permanently disabled and unemployable. She tells me that she has a short-term memory impairment and she has frequent seizures, which really scares me. All of my family members are Baptists and we have strong religious beliefs, so I know God will get us through this. My daughter has tried to work for short periods of time, but has been unable to do so because of severe memory problems.

Before the accident, my daughter was a very good girl; she had a great job and her own apartment and she was dating. (The man eventually left her after the accident.) She was also involved in gospel singing at her church. Now all my daughter can do is help me around the house. My other daughters come over quite frequently to see us, and I think they are resentful of her because they had to move out when she left the hospital. Because of my sickness, I was unable to manage all of them under the same roof.

None of the family members believe that my daughter was at fault for the accident, though they all wonder why she was not wearing her seatbelt at the time. I remember telling her the morning of the accident that she should always wear her seatbelt, even if she were driving close to home. If she had done all of this, this accident might not have happened and she would not be limited as she is now, but I guess we all truly believe that the accident had just happened and not for any reason. Regardless, all of us know that she was such a good person before the accident. We were very impressed with her lifestyle — a nice apartment with fine furniture and plants everywhere. In our eyes, she was a successful, yet quiet person. Now after the accident she is thinner and even more energetic. Yet I don't say "energetic" in a positive sense. She really has changed for the worse. I still think my daughter is attractive, hopeful, caring, and friendly, but my other daughters think she is more irritable and even a troublemaker. They think that, though she is not the youngest, now she acts like she is the baby in the family. My injured daughter does not share in these beliefs; she feels that she has not changed that much, though she does realize that she is more dependent on all of us, and she has even said that she is less attractive now. After living with my daughter now for several months, I don't think she is going to change too much. We all hope that she will get much better, but I wonder about that.

The most stressful part of our family life now is living with the seizures. We just can't do anything about them, and I worry that they might be fatal and that I might have a heart attack because of the stress. When I get upset, I get chest pains. When we are all here and she has a seizure, we pray together that she will come out of it. Though we panic, we know enough to roll her over from side to side to keep her from swallowing her tongue. Because these seizures happen, and I have a hard time managing them, my daughters come over often just in case. I do get a "funny feeling" when a seizure happens, and I had that feeling the day of the accident. I expect the seizures will get worse, and I don't know what I can do about it. But my many friends and my church have been a support to me during this trial.

Deep down I think it is good for me to have my daughter at home. My friends also seem to visit often. I am happy if my children are all right, and right now I am not so happy because of this brain injury business. I believe that families should take care of each other. I took care of my mother when she was dying and I expect my children will take care of me just as I cared for them. I can manage if we have this togetherness. The doctors are necessary, but it is family that really counts. Though these seizures, are getting the best of us, we just group together and do the best we can. God will take care of us.

Discussion questions on the personal statement

1. Whose "fault" was the accident?
2. Is it more difficult to let go of a "productive" pre-injured person?

3. What are the issues generated by wearing and not wearing a seatbelt?
4. Why are the seizures a source of stress?
5. What are the future concerns in the situation?
6. How can a religious perspective be helpful in coping with a brain injury?
7. How is a sibling's perspective of a head-injured brother or sister different from that of a parent's?
8. What are the advantages and disadvantages of being a single parent coping with caregiver responsibilities?

Set 10. Enough is enough

Perspective

An often overlooked factor in addressing the needs of the person with a head trauma and his or her family is the impact of additional illnesses on the patient and other family members and/or primary caregivers. This can be a major issue because the resources of the support system can be greatly stressed. An example of this would be the following case overview:

Sandra was a 45-year-old wife and mother of four children when she sustained a brain injury. She had lived a very active, vigorous life and was the central figure in her family system. Caring for and managing Sandra was facilitated by the commitment of her husband, Vernon, who felt it was a privilege to care for his wife and best friend. Although their children were living in the same town, they were able to maintain their separate lives due to the commitment and investment of their father. A major crisis occurred when their father suffered a severe heart attack and was in need of complete care himself. A temporary plan was to have an unmarried daughter move home to stabilize the situation. This worked for 3 weeks, until the daughter suffered a severe back injury while trying to lift her mother off the floor.

Faced with a decision to either place the mother in a nursing home or have her move in with one of the children, the family was forced to realize that they had to become involved at a higher level of commitment and personal sacrifice. This decision never had to be made because both the mother and father died within a month. This case overview illustrates two several points: first, viable caregiving arrangements can suddenly change, and second, multiple illnesses can have a synergistic effect, overwhelming the resources of both caregiver and family.

Exploration

Having read the above case synopsis, list other additional factors which could have further complicated this case.

1. Can you think of a family challenged by brain injury who had to deal with the impact of multiple illnesses? What was the outcome? Were there any intergenerational issues? What would have been helpful?

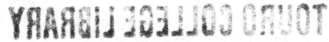

2. What are some areas of competence that are important for families challenged by a brain injury?
3. Who in your family would be able to shift roles and adapt to the changes caused by a brain injury?
4. What are the assets and limitations of being involved with a self-help group?
5. Do you think that families can ever be normal again after a brain injury?
6. Identify those extended family members who would not be helpful to you or your immediate family. State why.
7. If you are married, discuss how the severe brain injury of your spouse would change and challenge your relationship. How would you treat your spouse? How would your spouse treat you? How has your spouse responded to prior crises and losses?
8. What are the major life problems your family has experienced?
9. Have these problems existed from generation to generation?
10. How does your family handle bad news?
11. What are the needs of your family that have never been met?
12. How much help would your family need to cope with a brain injury?
13. How do you handle helplessness?
14. How does your family handle helplessness?
15. If your spouse was severely head injured, would you get a divorce?
16. If your spouse had AIDS, as well as a brain injury, what would you do? What would you need?

References

Barker, L. (1988) Newsletter, 8(3), 2, National Brain Injury Foundation, in Zeigler, E.A. (1989) The importance of mutual support for spouses of brain injury survivors, *Cognit. Rehabil.*, 7(8), 36.

Bullook, R., Chestnut, R., and Clifton, G. (1998) Guidelines for the managment of severe head injury, Brain Trauma Foundation, New York.

Coppa, C., Hepburn, J., Strauss, D., and Yody, B. (1999) Return to home after acquired brain injury: is the family ready?, *Brain Injury Source*, 3, 18–21.

Dombouy, A., Meirowsky, A., and Weiss, G. (1997) Recovery and rehabilitation following traumatic brain injury, *Brain Injury*, 11, 303–318.

Hart, T. and Jacobs, H. (1993) Rehabilitation and management of behavioral disturbances following frontal lobe injury, *J. Head Trauma Rehabil.*, 8(1), 1–12.

House, J.S. (1981) *Work Stress and Social Support*, Addison-Wesley, Reading, MA.

Jacobs, H.E. (1984) The family as a therapeutic agent: long-term rehabilitation for traumatic brain injury patients, *National Institute of Handicapped Research Report*, Washington, D.C.

Keydel, C.F. (1991) An exploration of perception and coping behavior in family members living with a closed head injured relative, Doctoral dissertation, University of Maryland, College of Education, College Park, MD, unpublished.

Leathem, J., Heath, E., and Wooley, C. (1996) Relatives perceptions of role change, social support and stress after traumatic brain injury, *Brain Injury*, 10, 27–38.

MacFarlene, M. (1991) Treating brain-injured clients and their families, *Fam. Ther.*, 26, 13–30.

Marmé, M. and Skord, K. (1993) Counseling strategies to enhance the vocational rehabilitation of persons after traumatic brain injury, *J. of Applied Rehabil. Counseling*, 24(1), 19–25.

Medlar, T.M. (1993) Sexual counseling and traumatic brain injury, *Sexuality and Disabil.*, 11(1), 57–71. Pieper, B. (1991) Injury and response: what parents and professional providers are telling us about treating children with traumatic brain injury, New York State Head Injury Association.

Pieper, B. and Singer, G. (1991) Model family professional partnerships for interventions in children with traumatic brain injury, New York State Head Injury Association.

Rosenthal, M., Dijkers, M., Harrison-Felix, C., Nabors, N., Witol, A., Young, M., and Englander, J. (1996) Impact of minority status on functional outcome and community integration following traumatic brain injury, *J. of Head Trauma Rehabil.*, 11, 40–57.

Sachs, P.R. (1991) Treating Families of Brain Injury Survivors, Springer, New York.

Treischmann, R.B. (1974) Coping with a disability: a sliding scale of goals, *Arch. of Phys. Med. and Rehabil.*, 50, 556–560.

Zeigler, E.A. (1989) The importance of mutual support for spouses of brain injury survivors, *Cognit. Rehabil.*, 7(3), 34–37.

chapter seven

Group counseling: a resource for persons and families challenged by brain injury

Perspective

Group counseling is a powerful intervention and resource that can help families coping with brain injuries.

When group counseling is applied to brain injury treatment and rehabilitation, it can become a counter-force to helplessness, isolation, and desperation. Group counseling brings people together to share their individual concerns, develop their resources, learn from each other's successes and failures, and establish a common ground for the rigors and demands of the treatment and rehabilitation process.

A major contribution of group counseling when applied to brain injury treatment and rehabilitation is that it provides an opportunity for people to explore the dimensions of their experiences and needs while developing skills to maximize their resources through a peer-oriented and goal-oriented support system. Group counseling can: 1. help put brain injury into perspective; 2. facilitate the development of resources; 3. support both the client and the family during the process of treatment and rehabilitation; 4. expose individuals and families to role models; and 5. teach the necessary skills to effectively respond to past, present, and future concerns.

As a result of the demonstrated value of groups with families and individuals, group counseling is becoming an integral part of treatment and rehabilitation (Ben-Yishay and Lakin, 1989; Campbell, 1988; Cicerone et al., 1997; Delmonico et al., 1998; Hopewell and Jackson, 1995; Hegeman, 1988; Jarman and Stone, 1989; Moreci, 1996; O'Neil-Prozzi et al., 1999; Rosenthal, 1987; Sanders et al., 1999; Schultz, 1994; Weisman-Hakes et al., 1998; Zeigler, 1989).

Critical issues related to group counseling with families experiencing brain injury

There are many consequences of a brain injury experience that can intensify the trauma and deplete personal and family resources. Some of these consequences are:

1. Marital relationships can begin to deteriorate, and spouses may see separation, resignation, or divorce as the only way to save and remove themselves from a situation they cannot handle (LaPlante et al., 1996; McLaughlin and Schaffer, 1985; Zeigler, 1989).
2. Siblings may react as a result of the changes in the family and they may experience resentment, jealousy, and parental pressure (Orsillo et al., 1993; Waaland and Kreutzer, 1988).
3. Substance abuse of a family member may develop as a means to cope with the stress and losses associated with a brain injury (Delmonico et al., 1998; Waaland and Kreutzer, 1988).
4. Work performance of the injured family member may deteriorate and result in loss of job (Jacobs, 1988; Witol et al., 1996).
5. Individual family members, as well as the family as a whole, can neglect themselves both physically and emotionally by not tending to individual or mutual needs (Hegeman, 1988).
6. Financial pressures can be seen as a cause of disharmony when, in fact, they may be symptomatic of underlying stress that is more difficult to concretize. DeJong et al. (1990) stated: "The costs of medical care, personal care, supervision, residential care and respite care for a person with a brain injury can quickly exhaust the financial capacities of even the most prosperous families" (p. 13). While focusing on financial costs, the authors make reference to the emotional costs and the similar depletion of emotional resources that can also occur.
7. Traditional support systems, such as friends, peers, and relatives, may remove themselves from supporting roles because of their inability to respond to the emotional demands made upon them (Armstrong, 1991; Jarman and Stone, 1989; Weisman-Hakes et al., 1998).
8. Educational goals and career opportunities may be altered, changed, or lost.

The challenge of group counseling is to address these concerns, manage a complex reality, and provide families with a structure and process to control their reactions while developing their resources. One of the most powerful insights that can take place in a group is the awareness that group members are not alone and that there are others who can help them to process what has happened and help prepare them for what will occur.

The importance of groups is discussed by Rosenthal (1987) when he states:

> ... groups offer opportunities to share common experiences, problems, and solutions; vent frustration and anger; and provide emotional support. Often, family members obtain specific information about community-based resources that can aid their relative (p. 56).

Cicerone et al. (1997) focus on the potential of groups:

> Group psychotherapy can be a valuable component of counseling for clients with traumatic brain injury. Group therapy provides a means to place the client in social situations, and therefore more closely approximate the demands of real life. This can serve to reduce the client's social isolation, and at the same time demands a broader repertoire of social and interpersonal behaviors ... . For some clients, sharing experiences with other persons who have a traumatic brain injury is a powerful form of alleviating the sense of alienation and demoralization (p. 36).

In a group, members are able to participate in an unfolding process that gradually prepares them to face and adjust to their loss and put in place the behaviors that will enhance the conditions for stabilization, gain, and growth. In a sense, it is an opportunity to interact and share with people faced with similar losses who can still cope and manage their lives, as well as learn from those who may not be as successful.

Group leadership and brain injury

Leaders of groups working with families living a brain injury experience must be highly skilled. They must have a broad perspective on brain injury, possess group leadership skills, be personally integrated, and have the ability to cognitively and experientially appreciate the impact of brain injury, loss, and trauma on the person and on the family.

The following is a list of some of the characteristics and skills that can be helpful to the role and functioning of a group leader:

1. Humaneness — an appreciation of the plight, struggle, needs, fears, nightmares, hopes, and dreams of families, which manifests itself in a caring kind, empathetic, and helpful manner.
2. Compassion — the ability to feel in a constructive and helpful way.
3. Resiliency — the ability to continue with the tasks of one's role in spite of personal emotional drain that often accompanies a repetition of "failure" or "no gain" experiences or personal loss which may be consequent to brain injury treatment and rehabilitation.

4. Intervention skills — ability to design and implement programs and responses that are timely, creative, visionary, and relevant to the evolving and changing needs of the person and family.
5. Medical knowledge — the ability to comprehend the complexities of a brain injury and secondary conditions and their impact on the patient, the family, and the group process.
6. Communication skills — the ability to relate to person, family, significant others, and members of the interdisciplinary health care team.
7. Ability to differentiate between individual and family problems.
8. Awareness of the energizing or synergistic effect brain injury and other situations can have on the group process, the individual, and the family system.
9. Ability to orchestrate group process with complex themes, e.g., other life losses including illness and disability of significant others.
10. Awareness of the independent and conjoint functioning of family subsystems.
11. Ability to be proactive rather than reactive.
12. Ability to work with a co-leader, who can be helpful with large groups and provide a mutual feedback and support system.
13. Ability to resolve personal, cultural, and ethnic prejudices related to appreciating the potential and liabilities of clients and their family members.
14. Cognitive and experiential awareness of brain injury and its consequences. Group leaders should have experienced a training format which focuses on what brain injury means to the person and the family. The ideal is to have a co-leader who has personally experienced the reality of a brain injury within their family. However, personal experience alone is not adequate, just as a professional degree does not always equate with effectiveness.
15. Comprehensive understanding of a model that is relevant, applicable, and useful to families challenged by brain injury who are engaged in a lifelong journey and not just a destination.
16. Understanding and appreciation of the intergenerational impact of loss, illness, and disability and how these can influence family functioning.

While group leaders should have at their command a variety of skills, resources, and perspectives, a group model can be more responsive to complex needs if it is comprehensive, proactive, and multidimensional. The need for a multidimensional model is reflected in a statement by Holmes et al. (1990) in a discussion of the role and contribution of mutual help groups to the rehabilitation process. They state:

> Mutual help groups typically provide members with
> a variety of services aimed at helping them achieve
> specific goals. Specific services can include transporta-

tion, employment information and education, disability education and service information, family and individual social support, daily living skills training, peer counseling, community exploration, personal advice, planned entertainment, self-advocacy training, help with problem resolution and financial information (p. 21).

Multi-dimensional group model

A viable group counseling model must go beyond a token response to the needs of families and individuals living with brain injuries. This can occur when a group counseling program addresses issues encountered and anticipated during the treatment, rehabilitation, and life and living process.

A multi-dimensional group counseling model for persons with brain injuries and their families should be designed to be comprehensive and proactive. A comprehensive proactive group model is one that

1. Is available throughout the brain injury experience
2. Has the potential to be adapted to a variety of settings (e.g., community, home, hospital, independent living, or rehabilitation facility)
3. Is flexible in meeting the evolving and changing needs of the person and the family
4. Can be fully integrated into a rehabilitation program
5. Is capable of transcending the hospital environment and meeting the demands faced in the community
6. Has didactic components to teach the skills needed to respond to a range of medical and nonmedical problems related to the brain injury experience
7. Can respond to other life losses, e.g., secondary illnesses that may play an important role in adjustment to the brain injury experience
8. Is capable of anticipating problems rather than just reacting to them

With a multidimensional group model, the needs of the families can be better met by providing a system of alternatives as well as supplementary groups which emerge from and are related to the family group. The family group is the central, core group, focusing on family issues. It is from this group that the other groups evolve and are connected.

The following is a list of potential subgroups and their focus.

- Peer Group — Focuses on needs of the person in a group setting with peers
- Female Group — Addresses role issues which are relative to female issues and concerns
- Male Group — Addresses role issues that are relative to male issues and concerns

- Children's/Sibling Group — Opportunity for children to share feelings and learn how to respond to their unique situations (e.g., the injury of a parent or the stress related to a sibling in a coma management program)
- Spouse/Marital Group — Concerned with nurturing and maintaining a realistic marital relationship while coping with brain injury, the importance of which is stated by Zeigler (1989):

> Spouses of brain injury survivors face particular problems which are often not addressed in brain injury family support groups. These issues can be effectively dealt with in mutual support groups. Since the number of spouses affected by brain injury is less than the number of parents who are affected, the availability of spouse support groups is limited. These groups do seem to be emerging in various parts of the country utilizing a variety of formats (p. 37).

- Caregiver and Significant Others Group — An opportunity to involve those persons who are a part of the families' or clients' interactional system (Armstrong, 1991)
- Didactic Group — Provides information and teaches relevant skills related to living in spite of a brain injury (Wiseman-Hanks et al., 1998)
- Theme Group — Permits the addressing of various issues related to the brain injury experience, e.g., parenting (Singer et al., 1994), education, sexuality, and substance abuse
- Medical Staff Group — Opportunity for health and human care workers to discuss issues related to their individual functioning and to provide a professional support system
- Educational and Vocational Rehabilitation Group — Addressing issues related to education, employment, and careers
- Life and Living Group — Focusing on the process of developing a quality of life and living in spite of and in concert with a brain injury

While these are some examples of potential subgroups, Hill and Carper (1985), in an article focusing on group therapeutic approaches with persons with brain injuries, identified a variety of other groups offered in a rehabilitation facility. The groups offered included: 1. speech-language; 2. education; 3. recreation; 4. occupational therapy; 5. nutrition; 6. psychotherapy; and 7. physical therapy. While recognizing that there are advantages in group work with persons who have had a brain injury, Hill and Carper (1985) state: "The use of groups for cognitive rehabilitation can offer motivation, new learnings and socialization for patients" (p. 26).

However, it is important to recognize that group counseling is not a magic solution to all the problems, concerns, and needs of this population. For some individuals, group settings may not be appropriate due to the nature and complexity of their limitations. In such situations, the criteria for group intervention must be whether or not a group will be an additive to a person's life and living experience.

Conclusion

Group counseling is a valuable resource in working with the family and person living a brain injury experience. A comprehensive, relevant, and available group counseling program is a means to

1. Expose families coping with brain injury to role models who were able or are trying to meet the life and living challenges posed by the brain injury of a family member
2. Provide a support system that will respond to the evolving and changing long-term needs throughout the brain injury experience rather than be limited to the concerns associated with acute care
3. Create a structure within which family members can respond to their individual and collective needs and receive support, understanding, and encouragement from persons in similar as well as dissimilar situations
4. Introduce family members to other resources based upon the knowledge and expertise of other group members, avoiding the unnecessary strain and stress of individual families having to struggle for information that is already available [Valuable resources for such information are The Brain Injury Association and other national, regional, and local agencies (Appendix A and B)]
5. Teach families how to cope by developing proactive rather than a reactive response to problems that are common to life and living after a brain injury
6. Provide a structure for the introduction of medical knowledge that is relevant and helpful to group members
7. Establish a consumer point of view in a professional world and facilitate dialogue with health care and rehabilitation workers
8. Create a level of accountability for all who are involved in the treatment of persons with brain injury (a collective of families and significant others is often more aware of what should be happening compared with an individual family in a state of crisis)
9. Diffuse problems before they become overwhelming to the family or its individual members by exposing families to the problems and solutions employed by other group members
10. Enable families to share the common burden of brain injury rather than be fragmented by the desperation that is often a by-product of isolation
11. Personalize the treatment by processing information in a caring, structured manner

12. Develop the group as a referral source that can result in professional, personal, and social contacts, which are essential in coping with brain injury over an extended period of time
13. Understand that the existence of a group counseling program does not mean that all problems related to brain injury can be solved, but that critical elements in the brain injury experience will have a better chance of being attended to
14. Advocate for what should be rather than accept what is offered as a result of resource depletion consequent to managed care and managed cost

Group counseling with families and individuals challenged by a brain injury is a major resource in personalizing the health care system and providing a vehicle for support, skills, mutuality, sensitivity, honesty, caring, concern, and consistency which can facilitate the adjustment to living with the effects and realities associated with a brain injury. Rocchio (1998) captures the power of groups: "Families find groups very helpful in gaining insight into the long term consequences of brain injury, ways to recognize problems in advance of their becoming difficult issues, and sharing practical management strategies with other families" (p. 16).

The major contribution of group counseling is that people can share their pain and hope, while realizing that they are not alone. The following personal statement, *Better Than Being Alone, A Husband's Perspective* focuses on the need for significant others.

Personal statement

Better than being alone, a husband's perspective

The worst part of having my wife become head injured was the feeling that nothing like this has happened to anyone before. Here I was, 41 years old, happy, and content. I was healthy, my 39-year-old wife was successful in her business, and our children were all doing very well. Nowhere in my background had I ever been exposed to a major illness or even considered it happening to me or my family.

On a tranquil fall evening my wife sustained a severe brain injury when she was struck by a speeding car while walking our dog. Fortunately, a passing motorist saw the dog standing next to my wife who was lying on the roadside and immediately called for help. I was notified by the police and did not realize the seriousness of the situation until I was confronted with the reality of the emergency room. I realized that I was not prepared for the seriousness of the injury or realize what was in store for my wife, children, or family. The next 5 months were a blur. I was terrified, confused, and uncertain as to what to expect. My family and friends were supportive, but not helpful. They were equally in shock and were just as overwhelmed as I.

When my wife began rehabilitation, I was delighted that she had survived, but I was not sure I could cope with how she had changed or how to deal with an uncertain future. Fortunately, I met a woman whose husband had been injured and who was a member of a support group. After sharing our stories, she suggested that I join the group. I did, but with very mixed feelings.

First of all, I found it very difficult to talk to strangers about personal things. Second, I was not sure what to expect or whether or not it would be helpful. At the first meeting, I was surprised to see 11 other people who all had family members with brain injuries. Though some had children, siblings, spouses, or relatives, they all shared the common bond of being in a very difficult place and not wanting to have to deal with the situation.

During the next several group meetings, I mostly listened, observed, and talked about superficial things. I also began to read the literature that was available and to realize that there was a lot more to this brain injury situation than I realized or wanted to hear. As painful as it was, it was helpful to begin to realize what I was up against.

In time, I became more comfortable with the group and began to realize that some people were doing better than others. I also heard people talk about wanting to run away, get divorced, or make a bad situation better. This range of feelings enabled me to share my feelings and also to get support and understanding from a group of people who shared my common fears, as well as dreams. Also, it was helpful to realize that I had choices. There were things I could do or not do. This helped me realize that I did not have to be a victim.

My most difficult challenge was to realize that my wife may not get better; she could even get worse. This was very scary for me and it was helpful to see other group members who were able to keep their focus on the big picture and consider their own needs and those of their family. While the group did not directly change my situation, it gave me hope, support, and perspective. It also helped me to establish a network of people who helped me gain my bearings, helped my children, and made me realize that I needed a lot of help from my friends and that it was a lot better than being alone.

Discussion questions on the personal statement

1. What are the advantages and disadvantages of not experiencing serious illness and trauma?
2. Discuss how the circumstances related to the onset of a brain injury can help or impede familiar and personal adjustment (e.g., in this case, the fact that the hit and run driver was never caught).
3. In this situation, when should the family have access to a family support group?

4. Do you think that family groups should be limited only to individuals who have spouses or children who are head injured? What are advantages and disadvantages of having mixed groups?
5. Is it helpful to have group members be exposed to situations that are much worse or much better than their own?
6. How long do you think a support group should be made available to people with head injuries and their families?

Set 11. Common pain, mutual support

Perspective

A harsh reality of illness and disability in general and brain injury in particular, is that individuals and families are often abandoned, isolated, and left on their own. Group counseling can provide a helpful alternative for families challenged by a brain injury by providing structure, support, and resources at a time of ongoing crisis. When thinking about group counseling and self-help alternatives, it is important to recognize that some families are not accustomed to sharing feelings with strangers and may resist the group counseling experience. In such cases, gradual exposure to group members may create the needed bridges to help families find a common ground and become receptive to a group experience.

Exploration

1. List five ways group counseling could help you and your family adjust to living with the effects of a brain injury and other disabilities or illnesses?
2. If you had a brain injury, would you voluntarily enter a group? Why or why not?
3. What would be the most difficult aspect of group counseling for you as a group member?
4. What would be the most difficult aspect for you as a group leader?
5. Are there certain people with illnesses or disabilities you would not want to associate with?
6. List the characteristics of group members that make you uncomfortable.
7. If you could choose a group leader to lead a group for persons and families experiencing a brain injury, what would be ten characteristics you would like this person to have?
8. What are the characteristics of a group leader that would put you off?
9. Do you feel that you are fully functioning in your own life so that you are a role model for others?
10. Would this change if you became brain injured?
11. What is the ideal size of a group for persons with a brain injury?
12. Identify the most upsetting situation that could occur for you as a group member and as a leader.

13. How long should each group session be? How often should they meet?
14. Should people with disabilities and people without be in the same group? Why or why not?
15. Should persons with brain injuries be in a group with individuals who are living with AIDS, spinal cord injury, or mental retardation?
16. Do you prefer a group model that stresses structure or feelings?
17. What are the characteristics of a group experience that are important for persons and families living with a brain injury?
18. How long should a group experience last — weeks, months, years?
19. What are the advantages and disadvantages of having families coping with illness such as stroke, cancer, AIDS, etc., participate in the same group as families impacted by a brain injury?
20. Are there issues that should not be discussed in a group experience?
21. Should a family ever be excluded from a self-help or family group program?
22. Should groups be led by family members?
23. What are the advantages and disadvantages of "professionally" led groups and groups led by survivors?
24. From your perspective, what is and should be the primary goal of group counseling for families who have experienced brain injuries?
25. Should the person with a brain injury always be part of the family group?
26. What are the disadvantages and limitations of a group counseling program for families living the brain injury experience?
27. At what point during treatment and rehabilitation should family members join a group?
28. Identify and discuss some reasonable expectations that family members may have of the group process.

References

Armstrong, C. (1991) Emotional changes following brain injury: psychological and neurological components of depression, denial and anxiety. *J. of Rehabil.*, June 15–22.

Ben-Yishay, Y. and Lakin, P. (1989) Structured group treatment for brain injury survivors, in Neuropsychological Treatment after Brain Injury, Ellis, D.W. and Christensen, A.L., Eds., Kluwer Academic Publishers, Boston.

Campbell, C.H. (1988) Needs of relatives and helpfulness of support groups in severe brain injury, *Rehabil. Nursing*, 13(6), 320–325.

Cicerone, K.D., Fraser, R., and Clemmons, D. (1997) *Counseling Interactions with Traumatically Brain Injured Clients*, CRC Press, Boca Raton, FL.

DeJong, G., Batavia, A.I., and Williams, J.M. (1990) Who is responsible for the lifelong well being of a person with a brain injury?, *J. of Head Trauma and Rehabil.*, 5(1), 9–22.

Delmonico, R.I., Hanley-Peterson, P., and Englander, J. (1998) Group psychotherapy for persons with traumatic brain injury: management of frustration and substance abuse, *J. of Head Trauma and Rehabil.*, 13(6), 10–22.

Ehrlich, J.S. and Sipes, A.L. (1985) Group treatment of communication skills for head trauma patients, *Cognit. Rehabil.,* 3(1), 32–38.

Hegeman, K.M. (1988) A care plan for the family of a brain trauma client, *Rehabil. Nursing,* 13(5), 254–259.

Hill, J. and Carper, M. (1985) Greenery: group therapeutic approaches with the head injured, *Cognit. Rehabil.,* 18–29.

Holmes, G.E., Karst, R., and Goodwin, L.R. (1990) Mutual help groups and the rehabilitation process, *Am. Rehabil.,* 19, 20.

Hopewell, C.A. and Jackson, H.F. (1995) *Family Support Groups: Traumatic Brain Injury Monograph Series,* Dallas Neuropsychological Institute, Dallas.

Jacobs, H.E. (1988) The Los Angeles brain injury survey: procedures and initial findings, *Arch. of Phys. Med. and Rehabil.,* 69, 425–431.

Jarman, D.J. and Stone, J.A. (1989) Brain injury: issues and benefits arising within a family support group, *Cognit. Rehabil.,* May/June, 30–33.

LaPlante, M.P., Carlson, D., Kaye, H.S., and Bradsher, J.E. (1996) Families with disabilities in the United States, Disability Statistics Report (8), U.S. Department of Education, National Institute on Disability and Rehabilitation Research, Washington, D.C.

McLaughlin, A.M. and Schaffer, V. (1985) Rehabilitate or remold? Family involvement in head trauma recovery, *Cognit. Rehabil.,* 3(1), 14–17.

Moreci, G. (1996) A model system of TBI peer support: importance, development, and process, *NeuroRehabil.,* 7, 211–218.

O'Neil-Prozzi, T., Flemming, K., Sanders, R. (1999) Efficacy of Individual versus Individual and Group Outpatient Therapies, Research Project #4, Spaulding Hospital, Boston,.

Orsillo, S.M., McCaffrey, R.J., and Fisher, J.M. (1993) Siblings of head-injured individuals: a population at risk, *J. of Head Trauma Rehabil.,* 8(1), 102–115.

Rocchio, C. (1998) The unvarnished truth, there is no cure for brain injury, *Family News and Views,* Brain Injury Association, Alexandria, VA, 15, 16.

Rosenthal, M. (1987) Traumatic brain injury: neurobehavioral consequences, in *Rehabil. Psychol. Desk Reference,* Chaplain, B., Ed., Aspen, Rockville, MD.

Sanders, R., Kaiser, R., and O'Neil-Prozzi, T. (1999) Efficacy of a group model for including family members in the treatment of the patient with TBI, TBI Newscaster Spaulding Hospital, Boston.

Schultz, C.H. (1994) Helping factors in a peer-developed support group for persons with head injury, *Am. J. of Occup. Ther.,* 48(4), 305–309.

Singer, G.H., Glang, A., Nixon, C., Cooley, E., Kearns, K.A., Williams, D., and Powers, L.E. (1994) A comparison of two psychosocial interventions for parents of children with acquired brain injury: An exploratory study, *J. of Head Trauma Rehabil.,* 9(4), 38–49.

Videka-Sherman, L. and Lieberman, M. (1985) The effects of self-help and psychotherapy intervention on child loss: the limits of recovery, *Am. J. of Orthopsychiatr.,* 55, 70–82.

Waaland, P.K. and Kreutzer, J.S. (1988) Family response to childhood traumatic brain injury, *J. of Head Trauma Rehabil.,* 3(4), 51–63.

Walwork, E. (1984) Coping with the death of a newborn, in *Helping Parents and Their Families Cope with Medical Problems,* Roback, H.B., Ed., Jossey-Bass, San Francisco.

Wiseman-Hanks, C., Steward, M.L, Wasserman, R., and Schuller, R. (1998) Peer group training of pragmatic skills in adolescents with acquired brain injury, *J. of Head Trauma Rehabil.,* 13(6), 23–38.

Witol, A., Sander, A., Seel, R., and Kreutzer, J. (1996) Long term neurobehavioral characteristics after brain injury: Implications for vocational rehabilitation, *J. of Vocational Rehabil.*, 7, 159–167.

Zeigler, E.A. (1989) The importance of mutual support for spouses of brain injury, *Cognit. Rehabil.*, May-June, 34–37.

chapter eight

Career, employment, and work issues

Because of improved emergency and acute care treatment, more individuals with closed brain injury survive each year (MacFarlene, 1999). Many of those who survive, however, may incur behavioral, cognitive, and physical impairments so severe that a return to independent living is impossible. Other survivors are able to live somewhat independently, though they may experience difficulties in daily living or returning to their former employment (Jacobs, 1988).

Traumatic brain injury (TBI) can often change the person's career direction in terms of the worker role and earnings lost (O'Neil et al., 1998). Many individuals, especially those for whom employment played both a vital role in their lives and was a substantial contributor to the quality of life, are willing to explore the possibilities of returning to work outside of the home, resuming another career, or at least be employed part-time. This chapter will focus on the career development of those who have experienced a TBI and express a willingness to explore career and work options.

Since most brain injuries occur during the teenage and young adult years when values are being learned which will eventually contribute to career success (O'Neil et al., 1998), school-based programs have been developed which focus on this population and provide retraining of important skills for work adjustment. The post-young adult population usually has access to community-based programs that emphasize cognitive retraining and work hardening. With all of these populations, the available family has an important role in the development of career choices or when one wishes to resume previous employment. This chapter will emphasize this family role.

Employment status after injury may be of crucial importance to the brain-injured person and his or her family. Inability to return to work can result in loss of earning power and long-term financial dependence. Loss of career possibilities leads, moreover, to the loss of both one's values as a person and economic options as well as loss of self-confidence. Because uncertainty of life usually associated with a head injury contributes to a loss of self-esteem, career planning conducted as soon as appropriately possible following the trauma may instill hope and even enthusiasm for a productive future. The family can create a climate for the injured person that may promote both eventual employment planning and generate the person's realization of some productive capabilities. Career decisions may be closely related to family dynamics. For example, family expectations express the family goal that every member will follow a career.

However, returning to work, or the development of a new career, may not be a feasible goal for the family member nor may it validate the family's view of themselves in relationship to work. Loss of income, the presence of secondary gains, and the willingness to maintain dependency are all factors that can inhibit career planning. The person with a TBI may simply not benefit financially from a return to work, and leisure or related avocational interests may have to be considered.

Family attitudes can make a difference for the young person in the development of a career identity. Career decisions by an individual with a brain injury may be the result of interactions between the person and his or her family (Lopez and Andrews, 1987). The family context of attitudes, expectations, and communication patterns may be a significant factor in determining career directions or whether one even wishes to explore return-ing to work or beginning vocational training. For adults with brain injuries, coping with any serious career disruption involves not only the use of family and interpersonal factors in planning, but also other environmental, eco-nomic, and medical treatment strategies.

Before explaining the family's contribution to the career development process, certain issues must be identified which provide a context for under-standing the role of the family. While success in the career arena can be expected to have a substantially, positive impact on a client's overall quality of life, this goal is not possible without a knowledge of realities that influence both the injured person and the family.

Career-related issues

There are several issues that must be considered when planning career development strategies with those who are brain-injured (Curl et al., 1996). Several of these factors interact with family dynamics and highlight the importance of involving the family in future employment planning.

Readiness

An injured person's age, sex, duration of loss of consciousness following the brain trauma, and extent of cognitive disorders can influence an individual's ability to resume an employment career (Cifu et al., 1997). Sustained neuro-logical injuries, as well as motor and ambulation deficits, can inhibit even the initiation of vocational-related interventions. Persons with significant psychological and/or emotional disturbances cannot reasonably be expected to be successful in the vocational rehabilitation (VR) process. More severe injuries are associated with poor vocational outcomes (O'Neil et al., 1998). Such psychosocial factors as denial of one's cognitive and behavioral limitations, the loss of pre-injury, acquired interpersonal relationship skills, and the reduction of learning ability may necessitate a delay in any planning efforts for the attainment of career goals. Personality problems inhibit career adjustment and the family member with a brain injury may simply not be ready for career exploration. If the person, moreover, has a history of poor self-concept and accompanying feelings of inadequacy, the trauma may intensify these feelings and reduce any motivation for employment planning. Family members can often inform health professionals of the client's behavior in the home, behavior which could suggest an inability at a particular time to adjust to work demands. An issue related to readiness of the person with brain injury is whether the family is ready for the member to return to work or begin career exploration. Family expectations for the person's eventual productivity may be quite different from those stated by health and vocational professionals. The family's fear of the future, intense concern for the individual's safety, and inability to understand a return to work or career exploration process may inhibit the willingness of the family to be involved in career redevelopment pursuits.

Available resources

For the brain-injured individual it may not be a lack of motivation or preparation to resume career opportunities. Vocational resources which could provide insightful information on how to build on the residual, career-related strengths of the person with brain trauma may not be readily available. VR as a service delivery model is a distinct and separate process apart from medical rehabilitation. This service delivery model includes supported employment, cognitive remediation, work hardening, and vocational assessment programs (Devaney et al., 1991; Powell et al., 1991). For some families, because of geographical location or socioeconomic levels, such services may not be accessible. Many families, moreover, are not aware that these career-related rehabilitation opportunities exist. Included among available resources are family competencies that can be used to meet career demands, as well as advocacy skills and the capability for understanding information on brain trauma.

Early intervention

If an individual who has incurred a brain injury is to eventually resume an occupational career, then early intervention is a necessity. Early intervention implies that as medical rehabilitation is conducted, the client and family are informed about possible services, and information is conveyed to these persons when appropriately possible concerning those residual capabilities which can establish the foundation for career building. If the family is to be an effective partner in their member's VR efforts, then when there is some degree of stabilization of medical problems, information needs to be communicated to them about career expectations and how to explore the resumption of career possibilities. If early intervention is initiated with the family, a family assessment can be conducted (as explained in Chapter 5), focusing on the exploration of such issues as the family's willingness to be involved, past and present coping strategies with any family crises, cultural beliefs, family expectations, and available social support resources.

Skills of the professional

Though VR is a distinct process from medical interventions, those who deliver these latter services need to be knowledgeable about career-related opportunities and how they can communicate them to the client and family (Ninomiya et al., 1995). It is important for career planning that families understand the nature of the VR process, what to expect, and how each member of a rehabilitation team contributes to the achievement of work-related goals. To convey this information requires both awareness and skills. For example, career services should not be initiated without adequate attention to how problems in the client's cognitive and behavioral deficit areas influence career adjustment. The client should have the necessary pre-requisite skills for involvement in VR. These skills embrace the cognitive, emotional, and behavioral areas so that the client can learn new tasks, adjust appropriately to interpersonal situations, and follow instructions. It may not be necessary to wait for a resolution of all medical problems. The professional should have the skills to determine when career planning can be introduced, what reasonable accommodations should be made during any vocational training, and what career goals appear to be feasible. In other words, professionals should discern whether observable deficits can be resolved or what will interfere with or cause a failure during the VR process. Many deficits can be managed by work-site modifications or restructuring of work responsibilities (Johnson, 1987). There is also a need for medical professionals to connect with other professionals who may be more directly involved with VR tasks. An integration of medical services with VR services can contribute to a more appropriate and efficacious achievement of career goals. Because of such integration, the client's options for career opportunities can be expanded. Alternative forms of employment emerging from medical and vocational assessment may be more feasible for many with brain injuries. These options are usually the results of close coordination among all members of the individual's rehabilitation team.

Interactional nature of career decision-making

The family can create a climate that could promote career decisions. The interactional connection between family members which expresses openness, frankness, support, and the communication of positive expectations to the family member with a head injury can produce a career outcome that reflects a larger set of transactions between the brain-injured person and the family (Lopez and Andrews, 1987). Career development and family dynamics are closely linked. These links will be explored in the next section of this chapter.

Career development of those with brain injuries

The focus of this section is on the family's role in facilitating the career development of the individual with a TBI. Family dynamics and career exploration and adjustment are not two distinct spheres bearing no relationship to each other. There is a functional inter-relationship between the two areas, and career options are developed generally as a result of the interplay between the individual and the family. Moreover, career development for many who are brain-injured is actually a redevelopment or recycling of work goals, motivation, behaviors, and competencies (Sample and Rowntree, 1995). The family provides a context for this career process.

The theoretical framework that will provide a structure to understand both the stages of career development and the interaction with the family and the individuals during this development is taken from Hershenson's (1981) model of disability and work adjustment (Hershenson and Szymanski, 1992). Many models have been developed to explain why an individual has made a specific career decision, or how career satisfaction is achieved from the fit between a person's personality, characteristics, and abilities and career characteristics found (Holland, 1973; Krumboltz, 1979; Super, 1990; Astin, 1984). All of these approaches emphasize that career development is a continuous process over the lifespan and this development involves both career choice and career adjustment issues. Those with a TBI are usually faced with redeveloping their energies, residual abilities, and interests to more realistic, achievable career goals. The trauma represents a life disruption, and for those who are able to resume a prior career or explore new opportunities, a process begins that requires coordination between medical personnel, vocational counselors, and family members.

Hershenson's model (1981) does not explicitly include family dynamics, but it provides a useful framework to understand what should be addressed during the career development process and what is needed to achieve career goals, including return to work. Note that while Hershenson uses the term "work" throughout his explanation of his approach, these authors substitute the term "career," a more comprehensive concept relevant to those who may not be able to return to work soon after medical rehabilitation but who need an extended period of time to engage in career exploration. Moreover, the model combines features of career development and work adjustment theories, and has been identified in the literature as particularly applicable to persons with brain injuries (Kosciulek, 1991). Because the two essential elements in this model are the person and the person's environment, it is readily adaptable for a family and can also suggest guidelines for family members on how they can assume active roles in the career redevelopment of the injured person.

For an individual who is attempting to consider the career process following a TBI, Hershenson (1981) has identified three domains: career personality, career competencies, and when appropriate, crystallized career goals. These domains are in an interactive relationship with each other and the family environment. The product of the interaction is career adjustment which includes appropriate career behavior, engagement in suitable tasks, and career satisfaction. For a person with a brain injury, the impact of the disability is initially on potential or actual career competencies. If previously acquired work competencies are retained or restored following an appropriate period of rehabilitation or if the personality of the injured person can minimize or compensate for the loss of competencies, career adjustment and goals can be achieved.

Each component of the model is now discussed, adding emphasis on how the family can facilitate the development of the career personality, career competencies, and career goals.

Career personality

As explained by Hershenson (1981) career personality is characterized by three factors — self-concept, motivation, and needs (Hershenson and Szymanski, 1992).

Self-concept

TBI is a major blow to one's self-esteem. The injury can affect cognitive and physical abilities and one can lose self-confidence in pre-trauma capacities. In turn, this loss impacts on how the individual defines himself or herself as a person. How much the self-concept is affected depends on the extent of the brain injury, the age of the person, when the trauma occurred, and how the trauma compromises accustomed coping abilities that may have been quite effective pre-injury. This loss of self-confidence inhibits the family member's initiative to return to work and it can even bring a sense of hopelessness to the career exploration process.

Family members, however, when understanding the nature of the brain injury loss and subsequent losses and when focusing on the residual capacities of the injured family member can provide a family environment that emphasizes appropriate hope for the future and a recognition to the family member that his role in the family does not have to radically change. Because a person may be impaired does not mean that the individual doesn't have skills that make the impairment moot in the workplace. If family members do not make incorrect assumptions about what the person can or cannot do and involve the person in as many family activities as appropriately possible, then these actions may help to convince the injured family member that he or she can be a contributor to life. Positive communication styles and shared involvement frequently emerge, however, from family expectations and coping strategies. The attempt by family members to stay as involved as possible in their family and community activities in spite of the brain injury impact on their life, is a useful coping tool and often sends the message to the injured that life must go on and that he or she is expected to be as productive as possible.

Career motivation

An interest in beginning the career exploration process or return to work can be ambivalent. Three groups of factors influence the motivation to return or begin career exploration: personal variables, such as the values of family members, success in pre-trauma work activities, and an orientation that work is integral to maintaining self-esteem; background variables, such as gender, age, and residual cognitive abilities; and environmental variables, such as support from family members, previous employers, and others who could provide assistance to reach career goals. Yet an awareness of injury-related cognitive, physical, and behavioral limitations and the realization that financial resources can provide for a reasonable comfortable life may deter a family member from any career redevelopment efforts. Research has suggested that the stronger the work motivation pre-trauma, the greater the frustration over career or work-related limitations post-trauma (Ezrachi et al., 1991; Fabiano and Crewe, 1995). This frustration inhibits the desire to reach career/work adjustment goals.

To restore a family member's interest, willingness, and energy to undertake activities that will eventually lead to restored career productivity demands family support and an active role in family life. The person with a brain injury must be aware of the need to restore a career, and how the gradual return to employment, when possible, can make a difference in the quality of family life. For some persons, however, career will simply mean a job. Because of cognitive limitations, a basic non-demanding routine job may be the most feasible employment goal. Messages that family members convey about the importance of a satisfying career, that job accommodations can make it possible to actualize career abilities, and that family support is readily available for the continued attempts to engage in and proceed through the career redevelopment process may trigger the person's willingness to pursue career goals. An individual is more likely to re-enter an occupation if he or she has been positively reinforced by a valued, family member who advocates the person's engagement in that occupation and/or has access to resources with necessary information (Krumboltz, 1979). Information available to family members on what is feasible concerning work-related capacities and which resources can provide assistance for the achievement of career goals, are usually necessary to restore the person's career motivation. Fear often impedes family members in becoming a resource for the person's career redevelopment, but information about the family member's employment strengths, as well as understanding of the community programs developed for career assistance, can alleviate much of the family's fear over possible career failures.

Career needs

Individuals successful in the pursuit of productive careers have control needs and desires for achievement, interpersonal contact, security, and helping others, and they achieve harmony between interests, abilities, and career opportunities. A brain injury trauma may cloud these needs, removing them from one's awareness until post-injury stability (Ip et al., 1995). Once stability has been gained, the individual with an injury should have some feedback on how career-related or specific job needs can be met. This feedback begins with a comprehensive assessment of career-related capacities and the communication of information on relevant, appropriate opportunities. The realization of a possible match between a person's career-related needs and feasible opportunities should be achieved by the injured person as early as possible post-traumata. Needs are often neglected during the career exploration process, but the perception that career needs may be satisfied through career redevelopment efforts can stimulate the client's motivation to begin looking at career options.

If such basic needs as interpersonal contact, security, and the helping of others can be partially satisfied in the family environment, this satisfaction can set the stage for the eventual realization of career needs. Families should be aware that their injured member is undergoing a dramatic transition from pre-injury emotional, physical, and intellectual functioning to an adjustment to appropriate life goals. An individual's needs do not change; in fact, needs for security, interpersonal contact, and a feeling of productivity can become even more pronounced post-TBI. The give and take of family interpersonal dynamics and the allowance of the person with a TBI to become involved in family responsibilities can help this person become more aware of personal strengths. This awareness is another impetus for career exploration. Work adjustment demands adequate interpersonal skills, the conviction that what one is doing is worthwhile, and the security emerging from safety and financial factors. This adjustment can begin in the home following in-hospital medical rehabilitation.

Underlying these three factors of self-concept, motivation, and needs are the family themes of expectations and individual coping strategies. If the family has the positive attitude that career redevelopment is possible, family behaviors will emerge from this conviction. Consequently, family members will focus on what the injured person can do and how he can contribute to the family, and any feasible career exploration efforts will be supported by the family. Support from within is also an effective coping style. A lack of support for seeking career opportunities can discourage the person's initiative for eventual employment-related training and work goals. When the family can constructively displace their frustration and disappointments, stay active in their customary duties, pastimes, and responsibilities, and minimize the perceived failures accompanying rehabilitation, these strategies become positive ways to manage the brain-injury trauma on the family. They generate an environment within the home which is positive for the person who is seeking to re-adapt his or her shattered life to more realistic opportunities for career productivity.

Career competencies

With career personality, the development and/or retraining of competencies will be necessary to achieve career goals. A strong career/work personality, moreover, may compensate for the loss of competencies since career goals can be revised to accommodate the new realities of physical, emotional, and cognitive limitations. Hershenson (1981) identified three career/work competencies, all of which are relevant to how the family can influence career-work habits, career-related physical and mental skills, and career-related interpersonal skills (Hershenson and Szymanski, 1992).

Career habits

Successful adjustment to the career-seeking process and to an employment situation demands accuracy in performing tasks, efficiency in using one's time, organizing an approach to accomplishing tasks, an ability to follow instructions, and a capacity to pace one's work. Many work hardening and adjustment programs focus on these areas in preparing someone for return to employment. Helping professionals are specifically trained in varied techniques to assist in making a suitable work adjustment. The family can be a useful partner in these training efforts. Once the family is aware of these resources and the person with brain injury is encouraged to enter an appropriate program, the family can become a partner by supporting the family member to take part in family activities and tasks. This participation establishes the groundwork for the development of work habits. The individual with brain injury may need assistance to appropriately pace his family responsibilities, to do the different tasks properly, and to organize his work so that tasks are done efficiently. Through gentle and patient assistance, different family members may help the person to re-adapt to the performance of necessary family responsibilities. This is usually a difficult challenge for family members, and even a delicate issue when the individual has been accustomed pre-trauma to independence and performing duties in a learned way, an approach that may no longer be feasible because of injury limitations. In this role persons in the family are not necessarily teachers, but partners with helping professionals who are undertaking work or career retraining.

It is important to consider that if an individual with a BTI is to re-enter the job market or begin career exploration, it cannot happen automatically. If an individual has been inactive within the home, any career/work adjustment is not going to be possible. Activities that take place within the home can be stepping stones and learning experiences to later activities, such as attention to task and the ability to appropriately regulate work output. These activities can also provide a person with brain injury insights into strengths and work-related limitations, and how to compensate for these limitations in an employment situation. Though it may be difficult for many with brain injuries to achieve a self-awareness of abilities and obstacles, this is an essential ingredient for the successful completion of the career development process.

Career-related physical and mental skills

For a person with a brain injury, the acquisition of these skills may be very difficult because of physical and cognitive impairments (Greenspan et al., 1996). Limitations in following directions, learning new tasks, and remembering previously learned job functions will depend upon the nature and extent of the injury. Cognitive retraining and work adjustment strategies may minimize several of these limitations, but the individual may still have to make a number of accommodations when engaging in the career redevelopment process or directly seeking employment.

The role of the family in assisting a member to acquire such work-related skills depends upon their understanding of the person's career options. This information should be communicated by health care professionals when the residuals of the injury are somewhat stabilized and vocational assessment is conducted which identifies possible career and employment strengths. Usually the family has a minor part in actual retraining strategies, apart from communicating expectations for the person's eventual productivity and making any necessary changes in their daily routine so that the injured person can attend training sessions. If the family member is involved in activities and tasks in the home, this person can gain an awareness of work-related obstacles and strengths. Again, engagement in these home tasks becomes a pre-career training preparation.

Career-related interpersonal skills

Periods of irritability, difficulties in handling stress, bouts of depression, anxiety over ability to adapt to possible training demands, difficulties in following specific work-related instructions, and withdrawal from other people represent serious problems when attempting to adjust to a work environment or engage in the stages of the career redevelopment process. Anxiety and depression can inhibit career decision-making or self-understanding of potential abilities. Isolation from others can, of course, be a deterrent to any appropriate work adjustment.

The interpersonal life of the family, however, can provide a context that will assist the person with a brain injury to redevelop such interpersonal skills as handling the stress accompanying interpersonal relationships, controlling irritability, and listening carefully to others (Leathem et al., 1996). Positive interpersonal skills integral to the communication styles of family members can have a modeling effect on the individual with a brain injury. If such skills are absent in family life, the family member may have a difficult time making the transition to the give-and-take of vocational training or work environments. Maintaining or creating a home environment that facilitates career-related interpersonal skills means holding the injured person to the same family communication standards and behavioral guidelines as other family members. Within the daily demands of family life, moreover, the individual can learn to adapt to any communication deficit and perhaps remediate serious problems such as isolation or unwillingness to cooperate with others.

Career goals

Appropriate career goals will emerge from self-understanding, the availability of feasible career options, and any intervention that links self-knowledge to viable career goals. Appropriate work goals are in harmony with a person's interests, self-awareness, and abilities. Crystallized work goals may be very difficult for a person with a brain injury to achieve. The presence of cognitive and behavioral problems or the episodic nature of these problems may cause occasional changes in work goals as the recovery process continues over a long period of time.

Through participation in family activities, however, the family member with a brain injury can gain a renewed understanding of his or her interests and work-related abilities. This involvement presumes that the family provides the time, opportunity, and support needed to make it possible for the person to become involved. Engagement also implies encouragement, communication of trust, and assurance of necessary assistance to accomplish needed tasks. What can also facilitate family member involvement are plans developed with the family by a rehabilitation professional which highlights different goals that could be achieved during at-home recovery time, resources needed for any family involvement, and obstacles to attain any goals. These plans should be formulated soon after hospital discharge, and when implemented in the home, become another step to eventual career planning and employment training.

Career personality, career competencies, and career goals are, therefore, key factors in providing a structure for any family involvement in the career, the redevelopment process, and the pinpointing of target areas for what is needed if the person with a brain injury is to achieve career/work adjustment. A balance must be maintained, however, between family participation and the injured person's autonomy. These factors, moreover, continually interact with the four stages of career redevelopment described in the next sections.

Stage 1. Assessment

The individual seeking career goals must explore his or her skills, values, and interests. These are characteristics of the career personality, and feedback gained through family activities and other opportunities, i.e., cognitive retraining and work hardening, can assist the family member in appreciating both the capabilities and obstacles for return to work or beginning of vocational training. A realistic assessment of a family member's career or work potential can also be a powerful motivator to begin career activities. Another focus of assessment should be the person's capacity for acceptance (Leathem et al., 1996). When the individual with TBI acknowledges injury-related problems and his or her behavior has been expressed through compliance with medical rehabilitation program routines and objectives and the endorsement of medical staff recommendations for career exploration, these factors can strongly suggest a return to work (Rehab, 1994).

Stage 2. Exploration

Following an understanding of residual skills, career-related values, and preferences for career choices, the individual can ask, "What options do I have?" An awareness of what options are feasible and available demands updated career information. Family members usually do not have this knowledge, but they can encourage health service professionals to identify where it can be obtained. Often, satisfying career re-development opportunities are lost because someone does not have accurate, comprehensive, and current information about training, job seeking, and appropriate career resources.

Stage 3. Goal setting and planning

At some point in the career redevelopment process the person with a brain injury must ask, "which career option is the best possible direction for me and my goals, and why is this the best goal for me?" Self-understanding of the person's career personality and competencies have a vital role in this decision. This decision-making process emerges from how the effects of the brain injury are perceived by the person and family members, what expectations the injured person and the family have for the achievement of career goals, and the level of support is available from family, friends, and community. The selected option can be perceived as the outcome of the transactions between an understanding of the person's values, skills, interests, career competencies and what is appropriate to target in the economy for work or career pursuits, and family dynamics. The nature of the decision can also provide a more accurate response to, "why is this the most suitable goal?"

Stage 4. Strategy

This final step in the career redevelopment process highlights the question, "how will I get to my goal?" This question preempts other queries such as, what specific behaviors are necessary to get there, when will each step occur, and who else is involved or needs to be involved? If the injured, the family, and the rehabilitation professional have formed a partnership early on in the recovery process, these shared responsibilities will assist the person to reach a feasible career goal. A person with a brain injury needs shared support to reach eventual career adjustment. Transportation and financial issues may necessitate a realignment of family roles and expectations. Partnerships and shared responsibilities conducted in the context of encouraging the person's independence are indispensable for the identification of needed career competencies and specific behaviors.

Conclusion

The ideas presented in this chapter do not exclude the importance of cultural influences on the family and their role in career development. How the brain injury is perceived, the role of the injured person in the family, how the family makes decisions, what family members expect of each other, the level of support received from friends and community, and how willing the family is to accept outside help are all issues that may differ among cultures (Lustig, 1999). Each family is unique and each family will have its own role in providing some form of assistance to a family member who is willing to explore career options. Underlying this exploration are the family's shared assumptions about their member's ultimate career-related productivity (Lustig, 1999). If these assumptions are known by family members and health professionals, this knowledge becomes an opportunity to establish intervention strategies that can assist the individual with a TBI to resume a career path again. The family is a driving force in supporting career goals.

Personal statement

The day my world turned
by Louise

My life changed on a Saturday morning in North Carolina. As a 46-year-old orthopedic surgeon, I was on my way to the hospital to see patients when suddenly the front end of my car was hit by a car going over 75 mph and driven by a young man who had been drinking. I was in the hospital for a week recovering from broken ribs, facial injuries, and a brain injury trauma. Once I arrived home, I had every intention of returning to my group practice. I had worked very hard to become a doctor and establish my practice, and I had achieved this also with the awareness that there are very few women in my specialty.

When I returned to work, I knew something was wrong. I was very tired, like something was constantly running me over. I planned in a few months for full-time resumption of my duties. I had spent my whole life getting to this point of an established medical practice. Divorced, I was supporting my two children because they had difficulty making it on their own. I bought a farm and they lived with me to help maintain the crops and animals. My hopes were strong about resuming my practice. I asked the plastic surgeon about one of my major mental complaints, keeping track of time, and he said that he'd seen a lot of brain-injured persons with that concern, but that usually this symptom was gone in 3 months. I thought, "Great."

When I was working in the hospital I used to have to keep track of 15 patients as well as their specific medical issues. I realized when I started back to work that I couldn't remember patients' names. I also couldn't meet the expectations of others. At home, I tried cleaning the bathroom and doing the wash at the same time, and I just couldn't do it. I don't know why. I was realizing that a total readjustment was needed in my personal and family lives. It was like throwing the family up in the air and wherever it landed, we would have to start growing together. Fortunately, all of us in the family wanted to grow together.

I found out that I couldn't remember what I read, and if there was a distraction I couldn't apply material read in the proper sequence. Unfortunately, I discovered that since I wasn't improving in an allotted time slot, I was beginning to be considered by other doctors as a malingerer. I was caught between being labeled a malingerer, which the head of my group practice actually called me, and not wanting to operate and take care of people because I couldn't keep track of what I was doing. I even forgot what I was seeing patients for. I'd walk into a room and call the patient by name and find I had the wrong chart in my hand and was calling the person by the wrong name. I made a lot of stupid mistakes which indicated something was not working right. I had very little motivation and no stamina. I bottomed out before I even started to work. All in all, it was dangerous for me to see patients. I received 75 percent of the audio and visual stimuli presented to me, but I processed none of it. I was also very slow in my reaction time.

As time went by, I realized it was not realistic to resume my medical practice. I believed the chances of regaining what I lost were probably not very good. I took a series of tests and Social Security found me totally disabled. My insurance company would not pay for several of my large medical bills during the first year after the initial trauma. I have medical insurance now, and I'm paying the premiums at a reduced rate.

I've found that most people don't understand head injuries, especially the medical profession. I look fine; I talk fine. Therefore, I should be able to act exactly as I did before the accident. But when I try to act like I used to, I fail. It's bad enough when you criticize yourself for not being as you were before the accident, but when society reinforces it, it's worse. You need a lot of support to help you through it. My intelligence isn't gone; I just can't access it. The general medical population doesn't understand mild to moderate brain injuries and the deficits that arise from them. This is very frustrating for me. It's scary that those who should have an understanding, don't.

Sometimes, I feel like going in the house, putting a paper bag over my head, and saying, "Hey, World, I want to get off." I don't mean to commit suicide, but to be a total hermit, because dealing with people is not a thing that can be regimented. I now have a lot of trouble dealing with people and I usually need to get away from them instead of seeking them out. Presently, I am going to a cognitive retraining program and working on the farm. Though I can't do anything consistently, I've realized that now, 2 years after the accident, I am still in the process of waking up. For example, I didn't realize for a year and a half after the accident that my house was dirty. I thought my house was immaculately clean. When I finally woke up 1 day and saw dirt, which had probably been there forever, I was totally amazed.

What has helped me now are many things. I really love music, dancing, and animals. Talking with groups of other head-injured people definitely helps because they understand and they'll say, "I didn't have that, but what I had was this." You realize that as a whole group, we have a problem. I realized early on that individually we all have deficits, but as a group, we are dynamite. We realize something that the general population doesn't, namely, that we all have deficits. Before you have a head injury, you don't think you have deficits. After talking, we came up collectively with a constructive way of doing things, and I've thought how wonderful it would be if hospitals could function that way.

I think I'm not ready yet for a new career. I'm still not totally awake. I can tell when I'm waking up. I just can't tell how much further I have to go. My waking up has come in stages. Yet I've always been a "can do" person, and I have to honestly face what I can't do.

Discussion questions on the personal statement

1. What are the losses presented by Louise?
2. Is the fact that she was injured by a drunk driver more impacting and problematic than if alcohol were not involved?
3. Was the 3-month statement of potential symptom relief helpful or problematic?
4. What is unique and challenging for a physician acquiring a brain injury?
5. Discuss Louise's statement, "I am still waking up."
6. Why has peer support been helpful?
7. What careers do you consider viable for Louise at this time?

Personal statement

Restarting my career
by Rosa

My husband, three children, and I were on our way to a summer vacation. We'd just left our house 10 minutes before when a car spun out in front of us on the highway. Several cars stopped behind us. The driver of a tractor trailer decided there wasn't enough reason for him to stop, so he tried to go alongside of us. He accelerated, but because there was a curve, his rig jack-knifed and hit all the cars. We were the last car in the chain and were hit in the rear. I was sitting in the back with the kids. My husband said, "Hold on," so I knew we were going to get hit. The kids were in carseats and I kind of held on to the handle in the car and laid across the kids. I was thrown up front and then back. My head, back, and neck went over the back of the front seat. I hit my head and my face was cut. I have three herniated discs and a disc that bulges on my spine. The fireman said it was good that I protected the children because the force would probably have broken their necks. The entire steel back frame of our car was ripped in half. I'm glad I did what I did, but I was told I probably wouldn't have been so injured if I had been sitting upright in my seat. My son still says, "Mommy, why did you lay on us?"

I was only in the hospital for a day, and the emergency room doctor released me and said to see my primary doctor and an orthopedist in a week. The X-rays did not show anything. My primary doctor sent me to an ortho-pedist, who gave me some medicine, and told me to do certain exercises. I chose not to take the medication because I was breast feeding. But something else happened to me.

The first night after the accident, I came home; I love to cook, but I couldn't cook. I stood at the sink for about 45 minutes and I couldn't figure out what to do first. I couldn't deal with the kids; I was starting to hit the children a lot. I couldn't drive if the window was open. I found my temper was explosive. I finally realized something was really wrong with me and nobody would believe me. I asked my husband to commit me and put me in the hospital. He refused to do so; I went to see a social worker, and my sister-in-law, who had been in a car accident, referred me to an attorney. He asked me to see another doctor — a neurologist, but my insurance wouldn't cover the visits. Finally I was diagnosed with a closed head injury. After I was tested, the doctor said it was not severe enough to warrant treatment. I was abusing my children. I'd lock myself in the bathroom and call my husband to say, "You've got to come home now, or I'm going to hurt the children." He'd say, "I can't leave work," and I'd answer, "Well, you can't leave the kids with me either." Now he feels he's the caregiver, which he really doesn't want to be. Right now we're trying to work it out. I don't think my husband wants to be with me. He said he stays because we have children and he feels guilty. I'm not the type of person he wants to love. My husband says that living with me now is like living with a stranger. We have run through our entire savings since the accident. My husband started drinking soon after the accident. He also travels a lot and is gone anywhere from 1 to 2 weeks a month. I have a troubled marriage. We have separated 3 times since the accident occurred 2 1/2 years ago. My husband has had a very good job, but dealing with all of this has been difficult for him. My mother and father who live nearby have been supportive. I have had many broken legs and other injuries, and they have always been there for me.

Before the accident I had a job in computer operations, holding a certif-icate in computer graphing. The accident was 5 days after I graduated from college. I realize that I have to get my career back on track. I go to cognitive retraining classes, which are helpful, but my field was computer graphics and it's taking a long time to produce work from my home. I do a newsletter for a non-profit agency. It used to take me a few hours to do a job like this, now it may take 2 days to finish the product. Before the accident I was in business long enough to know my capabilities and those of the computer, but now I really can't figure out what they are. I used to be well known for freelance graphic work, but the work must be done quickly, and now I fear I couldn't do it. I've said so when people called me. They don't call me anymore. Yet I still have the same work needs of money, fulfillment, and achievement. I've realized that any career redevelopment will have to proceed slowly. Strangely, one of my first tasks of relearning was starting our self-propelled lawnmower. It took me 1 1/2 hours to start it. I felt very pleased with myself and excited that I did it.

The problem I see with gradually using the skills that I have gotten back is that when I talk with people in the computer industry, I don't understand them. I don't want to talk to these people anymore because I feel like an idiot. When I do get a program in the computer, it's an accomplishment. The real career obstacles are people's opinions. I've been told that I should apply for Social Security disability, and I can't make myself do it.

Restarting my career will take a lot of patience. For me, career means all that I am trying to do in my family, like taking care of the children and my vegetable garden and being careful that I don't overload myself at one time with a lot of information. I also have to get my self-concept back. It doesn't help listening to people who are wallowing in self-pity, but it does help to be determined. It may take me longer to get things done, but I have high expectations for myself. I may become a receptionist. I wouldn't be happy with that, but it's a job making money, and paid employment would help my self-esteem.

I was always an active person, yet when your brain doesn't function half the time, it's very hard to keep going. Having goals is very important to restart your career. Another help is having someone believe in you. One of the women at my child's nursery school is an instructor and she said she'd be willing to help me in anyway she could. She knows about head injury accidents. To re-establish a career you have to remember a lot of things. This type of remembering is going to be very slow coming back. The best description I have of myself before the accident is that there are doers and there are watchers. I was always the doer. Now I feel very much like the watcher. I don't like that feeling.

Discussion questions on the personal statement

1. What is your response to Rosa's placing herself at risk to protect her children? What if they had been injured?
2. How would you respond to a mother who demanded that the family buy a new car with airbags, and as a result of a minor accident during which the air bag discharged, her child was brain injured?
3. Why are family members hesitant to believe that something is wrong with a loved one?

4. Should the potential for child abuse and substance abuse be considered areas of concern during treatment and rehabilitation? If so how should this be addressed?

5. Why is restarting a career complicated for Rosa?

Set 12. Loss of job, less of self

Perspective

Most relationships are based upon common goals, mutual respect, interpersonal concerns, and emotional and financial security. For those and a variety of other reasons, people choose to be with each other and enter a long-term relationship. Unfortunately, illness in general and brain injury in particular can introduce elements into a relationship that are stressful and challenging and the implications are overwhelming. Some relationships can negotiate their challenges while others struggle and erode.

Exploration

1. Think of a couple you believe has an ideal relationship. How would this change if one of them experiences a brain injury and results in their loss of career? Which one do you think could cope the best as a caregiver? As a patient?

2. If you know a couple who has successfully experienced a major trauma, discuss what enabled them to survive.

References

Astin, H. (1984). The meaning of work in women's lives: a sociopsychological perspective, *The Counseling Psychol.*, 12, 117–126.

Cifu, D., Keyser-Marcus, L., and Lopez, E. (1997) Acute predictors of successful return to work one year after traumatic brain injury: a multicenter analysis, *Arch. Phys. Med. Rehabil.*, 78, 125–131.

Curl, R., Fraser, R., and Cook, R. (1996) Traumatic brain injury vocational rehabilitation: preliminary findings for the coworker as trainer project, *J. of Head Trauma Rehabil.*, 11, 75–85.

Devaney, C., Kreutzer, J., and Halberstadt, L. (1991) Referrals for supported employment after brain injury: neurological, behavioral, and emotional characteristics, *J. of Head Trauma Rehabil.*, 63, 59–70.

Ezrachi, O., Ben-Yishay, Y., and Kay, T. (1991) Predicting employment in traumatic brain injury following neuropsychological rehabilitation, *J. of Head Trauma Rehabil.*, 6, 71–84.

Fabiano, R. and Crewe, N. (1995) Variables associated with employment following severe traumatic brain injury, *Rehabil. Psychol.*, 40, 223–231.

Greenspan, A., Wrigley, J., Kresnow, M., and Fine, P. (1996) Factors influencing failure to return to work due to traumatic brain injury, *Brain Injury*, 10, 207–218.

Hershenson, D. and Szymanski, E. (1992) Career development of people with disability, in *Rehabilitation Counseling: Basics and Beyond*, 2nd ed., Parker, R.M. and Szymanski, E.M., Eds., Pro-Ed, Austin, TX, 273–303.

Hershenson, D. (1981) Work adjustment, disability, and the three r's of vocational rehabilitation: a conceptual model, *Rehabil. Counseling Bull.*, 25, 91–97.

Holland, J. (1973) *Making Vocational Choices: A Theory of Careers*, Prentice-Hall, Englewood Cliffs, NJ.

Ip, R., Dornan, J., and Schentag, C. (1995) Traumatic brain injury: factors predicting return to work or school, *Brain Injury*, 9, 517–532.

Jacobs, H. (1988). The Los Angeles head injury survey: Procedures and initial findings, *Arch. of Phys. Med. and Rehabil.*, 69, 425–431.

Johnson, R. (1987) Return to work after severe head injury, *Int. Disabil. Stud.*, 9, 49–54.

Kosciulek, J. (1991) The impact of traumatic brain injury on work adjustment development, *Vocational Evaluation and Work Adjustment Bull.*, 24, 137–140.

Krumboltz, J. (1979) A social learning theory of career choice, in *Social Learning Theory and Career Decision Making*, Mitchell, A.M., Jones, G.B., and Krumboltz, J.D., Eds., Carroll Press, Cranston, RI.

Leathem, J., Heath, E., and Woolley, C. (1996) Relative perceptions of role change, social support, and stress after traumatic brain injury, *Brain Injury*, 10, 27–38.

Lopez, F. and Andrews, S. (1987) Career indecision: a family systems perspective, *J. of Counseling and Dev.*, 65, 304–307.

Lustig, D. (1999) Family caregiving of adults with mental retardation: key issues for rehabilitation counselors, *J. of Rehabil.*, 65, 26–35.

MacFarlene, M. (1999) Treating brain-injured clients and their families, *Fam. Ther.*, 1, 13–30.

Ninomiya, J., Ashley, M., Raney, M., and Krych, D. (1995) Vocational rehabilitation, in *Traumatic Brain Injury Rehabilitation*, Ashley, M. and Krych, D., Eds., CRC Press, Boca Raton, FL.

O'Neil, J., Hibbard, M., Brown, M., Jaffe, M., Sliwinski, M., Vandergoot, D., and Weiss, H. (1998) The effect of employment on quality of life and community integration after traumatic brain injury, *J. of Head Trauma Rehabil.*, 13, 68–79.

Powell, T., Pancsofar, E., and Steere, K. (1991) Supported Employment: Providing Integrated Employment Opportunities for Persons with Disabilities, Longman, New York.

Rehab, (1994) Community integration of individuals with traumatic brain injury, National Institute on Disability and Rehabilitation Research, 16, Washington, D.C.

Sample, P. and Rowntree, A. (1995) Employment intervention strategies for individuals with brain injury, *Occup. Ther. and Health Care*, 9, 45–56.

Super, D. (1990) A life-span, life-space approach to career development, in *Career Choice and Development: Applying Contemporary Theories to Practice*, Brown, D., Brooks, L., and Associates, Jossey-Bass, San Francisco, CA, 197–261.

part three

Issues and reflections

chapter nine

Loss, grief, and brain injury

Perspective

The occurrence of a brain injury can create, contribute to, or intensify a crisis in family life. It may also cause a family to enter a state of loss and complicated grief that is intense, consuming, and enduring.

Most family crises are usually temporary and are characterized by a search for immediate solutions that may or may not fit the families' resources or problemsolving skill set. However, when a family is engulfed by a brain injury, predictable feelings of desperation, depression, resentment, anger, grief, and sadness emerge. This state is frequently consequent to cumulative patient and family life losses which are magnified or intensified by the current crisis.

Placing the grief reaction in context of Parkes (1975) and Pollock (1961), Garner (1997) points out:

> The manifestation of any grief reaction is always influenced by a number of factors: by the previous experience of loss, the quality of the relationship and intrapsychic factors — ego strength and development, unconscious hostility, ambivalence and identification with the introjected patient into the self — all these contribute to the variation in the grief response (p. 181).

Attending to loss related to brain injury Gardner (1999) states, "Brain injury is almost always followed by loss of self esteem and unpleasant feelings e.g. depression, anxiety, guilt, shame, helplessness, powerlessness" (p. 8). This difficult emotional state can linger, expand, and cause a serious disruption to family functioning as well as impede family coping, caregiving, and recovery. At this point in time the family is at great risk.

This risk is addressed by Rosenthal et al. (1998) who state that families of traumatic brain injury (TBI) survivors, themselves, are at risk for depression and anxiety, and their level of maladjustment is associated with the severity of emotional changes in their brain-injured relatives.

While depression is often associated with the caregiving process (DeBoskey, 1996; Gallagher et al., 1989; Walker and Pomeroy, 1996), it is also a critical factor in psychosocial adjustment and social impairment related to traumatic brain injury (Gomez-Hernandez et al., 1997). Since depression often holds the family hostage, attending to its causes, consequences, and treatment is critical to facilitate and maximize rehabilitation and recovery.

Moldonado et al. (1997) emphasize this point:

> Depression may affect the prognosis of patients with primary neurological disease by preventing recovery, by accelerating the patient's deterioration, or by increasing the risk for complications. Depressed patients show greater impairment in the activities of daily living, cognitive functioning, and ability to participate meaningfully in rehabilitation programs yet it is both underdiagnosed and undertreated in neurological patients (p. 341).

Rosenthal et al. (1998) further address the importance of depression as a factor in brain injury rehabilitation:

> Depression is a barrier to the achievement of optimal rehabilitation goals in the successful reintegration of the patient into the home, family, community, and work environment. Thus, the accurate diagnosis, assessment, and treatment of depression after TBI is important for patients, family members, clinicians, and researchers (p. 90).

It is apparent that depression is a consuming and dynamic force that must be attended to in the context of both ordinary and extraordinary life experiences. Brain injury certainly qualifies as an extraordinary life experience.

Because depression, loss, and grief management provoke different intervention strategies and considerations, this chapter presents a perspective to understand, appreciate, and assist families engaged in a bereavement process related to a brain injury. Three areas are emphasized: 1. general considerations to be aware of when working with the family; 2. obstacles to effective grieving; and 3. interventions focused on meeting the family's current as well as future needs.

General considerations

Before connecting with a bereaved family, the health care professional should have an understanding of those factors and behaviors which will facilitate a helping approach that is relevant to the family living a brain injury experience.

Understanding the grief process

The importance of attending to grief and loss has been presented in a general context and a critical component in the health care process, especially as it relates to catastrophic illness and disability (Bowlby, 1980; Brown and Stoudemine, 1983; Doka, 1995; Fell, 1994; Heiney et al., 1993; Kubler-Ross, 1983; Miles and Crandell, 1983; Parkes, 1985; Rando, 1986; Reichley, 1995; Wright and Oliver, 1993; Zisook and DeVaul, 1985).

Grief is a powerful life force in shaping and influencing a family's experience with loss and change, which are the hallmarks of a brain injury. The challenge is for the family to cope with the loss of "what was" as it clashes with an altered and often unacceptable reality of "what is."

Grief responses by family members include emotions, thoughts, and behaviors that occur as a reaction to perceived family losses (Kane, 1990). Many losses are significant because of their symbolic meaning to the family (Brown, 1990). The perception of the importance of what has been lost affects the intensity and the duration of the grief. While grief is a normal and healthy reaction to loss, the strength and the duration of the family's grief response is often unpredictable due to a variety of life stressors — some known and others not anticipated.

Rocchio (1998) states:

> Problems developing after the individual is home and
> no longer involved in medical or rehabilitation settings
> may not be as readily recognized as a result of a brain
> injury and valuable treatment time can be lost if care-
> givers are unaware of some possible medical conse-
> quences of brain injury (p. 2).

When unanticipated or even predictable events occur, they can complicate the grief process by forcing the family to fight "several battles" concurrently. The war against brain injury can be lost by the cost of its many battles.

Kane (1990) identifies a four-stage process of grief as a response to loss. In this theory, grief resolution is an unchanging succession, and the activities of a stage are the ideas, emotions, and behaviors particular to it. These stages are 1. ignoring the loss; 2. experiencing the loss; 3. understanding the loss; and 4. changing with the loss.

Wright and Oliver (1993) state that children must accept the loss, experience the pain, and express their sorrow. They present children's reactions to serious loss or death as: fear, guilt, anger, and confusion. These are all intense emotions that can create distress for children and for families who may feel helpless to relieve the pain, replace the loss, or accelerate the mourning process.

Matz (1978) developed a lengthier descriptive model which captures many of the family's behavioral reactions, although families may differ in how they react to the loss. Matz believes that there are different stages of mourning in response to a traumatic event, and if a bereaved family is to reach an adaptive stage, family members will usually follow predictable steps in their grieving processes. The stages are:

1. "If I deny it, it's not true." The first response to a serious loss is usually denial, although Matz believes that the denial stage is "punctuated" by times of painful emotional awareness. The denial helps the family members to function and meet many of their daily responsibilities.
2. "I have the power to undo it." The denial gradually gives way to feelings of omnipotence. These feelings may be characterized by attempting to bring back the loss by searching efforts, or it may be expressed as anger at events or people the bereaved family regards as responsible for the loss. Unfortunately these efforts are doomed to fail, and gradually despair and helplessness occur.
3. "I can't do anything about it." Matz explains this as a time when the bereaved family members face the loss and begin to understand their feelings in order to reach an adaptive solution. The past may be reexamined, perhaps given up and partially replaced with hope. Depression also occurs, but hope may overcome it.
4. "I am rebuilding and every now and then I remember." The bereaved family members start to rebuild their lives. Social patterns are reestablished and new decisions are made to reach personal and family goals. According to Matz, painful memories will arise, but the family members appear to have more strength to deal with these emotions.

With all of these steps, however, the phases do not have clear-cut beginnings and endings. The move from phase to phase is gradual rather than sudden and dramatic.

Understanding intense grief reaction

Intervention approaches will differ between the family that has become overwhelmed consequent to the losses and demands associated with the brain injury experience and the family that is successful in maintaining its balance, grounding, and perspective. For example, when family members deny the loss, are evasive in their communication, show an absence of basic self-care as well as nurturing, and have persistent anger, guilt, hopelessness, and depression, they are displaying major adjustment problems. These will exact a toll over time and if not resolved may result in more difficulties and problems. This is often the case when families are so consumed by the crisis at hand that they are not vigilant and other problems and crises may occur which could have been anticipated or even prevented.

In contrast, the family that expresses an appropriate reactive sadness and begins to confront the reality of the brain injury may be better able to meet its responsibilities. Family communication styles are still intact. There may be some regression by family members to more childish, aggressive behaviors, but this is often temporary. Their sadness is actually a necessary part of the grieving process and the help provided to the family is mainly directed toward providing support for the alleviation of grief, encouraging hope, and providing support and access to role models.

Rando (1986) stressed the importance of comprehending the process of anticipatory grief and multiple losses that families have grieved in the past. This is an important issue because losses do not occur in a vacuum and they must be attended to in a familial, historical, and intergenerational context.

Reconceptualizing the needs of caregivers as involving losses that need to be grieved rather than just solved by general support or specific information represents an important change in direction (Walker and Pomeroy, 1996). This is a significant development in grief and loss resolution because it attends to the depth of the issue rather than focusing on surface manifestations.

Understanding the concepts of centrality, peripheral, preventable, and unpreventable

In a family system each member has a unique role that has a specific impact on family functioning. This is related to the importance of the person, his role, and his impact on family relationships.

Bugen (1977) explains the meaning of these terms as follows: if the person is central to family life, such as a loving parent or successful child, the loss will be greater than that associated with a person who is peripheral to the family. Whether the trauma was preventable or unpreventable will influence anger and blame associated with the intensity of the loss response. These concepts are important to understand because the health care professional frequently assists the family to move from a belief in preventability to a belief in unpreventability. It is important to note that many brain injuries, as well as other disabilities, are caused by the decision choices, action or inaction of family members, friends or significant others, and strangers. For example, many parents are burdened with the reality that they bought the bicycle (with or without a helmet) or car (with or without airbags) which was related to the brain injury of their family member. If the person is central and the family members are convinced the injury was preventable, then, as Bugen states, the grief will be both intense and prolonged. Initial intervention with the family will entail an assessment of the relationship of the impact of brain injury to the expectations, values, and beliefs of the family members.

Often those family members who reasonably adjust to the loss do so by drawing upon their resources and finding new meaning in living in spite of their family structure, dreams, and resources being greatly altered. This point is addressed by McKinlay and Hickox (1988) when they state "... severe brain injury may involve a loss of important qualities that were part of the person's premorbid personality. As with a true bereavement, role changes are often necessary" (p. 71).

Further, Rolland (1994) compares these second-order changes, which are "the altering aspects of one's world view and the basic rules that go with them" (p. 25), to first-order changes, which are the intensification of efforts within the boundaries of traditional roles such as gender roles.

Understanding the flexibility of goals for the family challenged by a brain injury

Families who are experiencing brain injury will have different needs. Many family members are looking for alleviation of the feelings of loneliness, isolation, and depression, whereas others are searching for a way to integrate the loss into family life. The challenge for families is to accept the loss, adapt to the loss, and try to assimilate the chronic sorrow into the family system. Stroebe et al. (1992) emphasize the need to let go in order to move on: "It might prove desirable to teach clients that there are many goals that can be set, many ways to feel and not set series of stages that they must pass through — that many forms of expression and behavioral patterns are acceptable reactions to loss" (p. 1221).

Kane (1990) emphasized that readjustment to loss and the achievement of positive change are dependent on coping capabilities, the family members' flexibility and adaptability, internalized locus of control, and adaptive skills. For the family expressing grief, intervention efforts are not only directed to alleviating the immediate pain but also to increasing the ability of the family member to change appropriately and cope effectively with a permanent loss.

Putting this in perspective, Stroebe et al. (1992) state:

> Grieving, a debilitating emotional response, is seen as a troublesome interference with daily routines, and should be 'worked through.' Such grief work typically consists of a number of tasks that have to be confronted and systematically attended to before normality is reinstated (p. 1205).

This is not an easy or simple process. In effect, families are often expected to deconstruct their world and redefine themselves in order to create a sense of purpose and meaning in their lives. The intensity of this process for caregivers living with multiple losses has been described as "the funeral that never ends" (Kapust and Weintraub, 1984, p. 462).

The common reality we all share is that certain events of the life experience must be accepted for what they are and that they are not always amenable to being molded into what we want and need them to be.

Knowing yourself as a health care professional

During bereavement, some family members may become extremely distraught. The health care professional may feel defenseless, uncomfortable, helpless, frustrated, anxious, fearful, and emotionally distressed. To experience anxiety and discomfort is normal, but for the health care provider or support personnel, these feelings can become so intense that they can hinder the helping process. In assisting the bereaved family, there is always going to be some agony, but if health care professionals have insights into their own defenses against grief and pain, many feelings of discomfort can be better managed and controlled. Consequently, more attention can be given to the needs of the family as compared to the needs of health care professionals. These can be addressed during professional education, training, or supervision.

The ability to listen, respond, provide support, impart information, and facilitate the familial exchange of feelings are skills needed by members of the health care team. These skills can assist families in coping with intense, profound, and often complicated grief.

To help families cope with loss also requires specific knowledge of the family, how its members perceive and handle grief historically and currently, as well as the ability to apply this understanding when family emotions are raging and unrelenting.

Stroebe et al. (1992) discuss the variation in forms of bereavement and advised researchers to be cautious about generalizing and considering "tailor made" treatments.

> Researchers might profitably be concerned with the enormous variations in the forms of bereavement ...
> This requires a highly sensitive receptivity — an open listening to the client voice for the reality and values of its sustaining subculture (p. 1211).

For most families the reaction to grief and loss is based upon what they have seen and learned. This family life experience is energized by the culture of the family which may not be familiar to the health care team or provider.

Obstacles to progress in grieving

With these considerations that represent areas of understanding for intervention in family loss, there are specific roadblocks to effective grieving. Brown (1990) has identified these barriers as described in the following sections.

Persistent denial of the permanent cognitive and physical losses

Family members continuously talk about "what was," and the past is continually reviewed or dwelled upon in order to maintain hope for full recovery and restoration of function.

Although the topics of death and dying are usually associated with bereavement, brain injury is an event that can cause intense family grief because it emerges from a pervasive sense of change, finality, and loss.

This loss is similar to other disabilities and illnesses that result in a major life transformation. Zemzars (1984) stated that for all chronic illnesses, the person can never fully return to his pre-illness state of health. This does not mean that gains cannot be made or goals attained; it does mean that in life we cannot stop time, each day we change and in that process there is a degree of irretrievable loss. This is due to the life altering impacts of traumas that transform the physical, emotional, and spiritual domains of a family's life.

The family's eventual realization that they and the family member will never be exactly the same can cause lingering feelings of deep sorrow. This point is made by Miller et al. (1994) who state, "Losses suffered by the debilitating effects of head injuries, stroke, or central nervous system dysfunction can be conceptualized as a partial death" (p. 50).

In contrast to a normative family crisis, which can be temporary or at least minimized through problem solving strategies, family loss and bereavement represent constant companions to family life. The grief, even though it may be diminished in its intensity or redefined with the passage of time, can be a pervading theme for intergenerational family life. For some families the losses of the past are active influences and forces in day-to-day life. They must be understood and addressed to create the conditions of healing and grief resolution.

Inability to express negative effect because of the loss

Bowlby (1980) explains that anger and crying are necessary responses which can lead to the recognition that the loss is final. The inability to cry or rave at the loss is often a consequence of society's dictates to maintain appropriate composure at the time of the loss. The initial grief response may also be inhibited because of a family member's fear of how a grief reaction may affect the injured family member or other members. Some families believe that the recognition or release of angry feelings associated with a loss is inappropriate.

Difficulties in dealing with ambivalence and feelings of resentment related to the loss

Brown (1990) reports that the closer and more positive the relationship with the lost object, the more difficult and prolonged the grief reaction can be. However, in some situations the loss may result in selected gain for the family or caregivers. For example, some families are pleased to have the member at home or in their care. Others are delighted to have the person leave home, to have minimal interaction, and to allocate their energy and resources in other areas rather than caregiving.

Unfinished business related to other losses

The current losses resulting from the head trauma may stimulate previously unresolved grief related to past losses which may have never been completely resolved, discussed, or understood.

Absence of limited coping skills or support network

Many family members may not possess adequate coping skills which can be accessed at the time of loss and they may not have the resources to develop them.

An intervention approach

When addressing a family's bereavement consequent to brain injury, emphasis is not necessarily on the immediate resolution of the grief but on assisting the family to function effectively as they understand how to manage and process their own sorrow, grief, and loss. A key point is to help the family cope in a constructive way and to avoid making the situation worse by poor decisions and maladaptive behavior.

This grief management requires specialized skills and perspective. The skills include the ability to access, create, and develop support mechanisms that inspire hope based on reality, but not limited to it. While reality can be a "common ground" for the family and the health care team, it can also be perceived differently. To the family, it can be overwhelming because they are engaged in a very subjective life experience as compared to the objective frame of reference of the health care team. The reality demands for the caregiver may be in excess of current or future resources. This can create a desperate situation.

Intervention should begin as soon as possible after the occurrence of a brain injury. This is dependent upon the family's needs, their readiness, and their ability to respond. In assisting a family it is important for the members to understand the source of their loss, then admit this loss and express their fear as well as their hope.

Nunn (1996) presents the importance of hope and its relation to the future:

> Hope, then, is that general tendency to construct and respond to the perceived future positively. The hopeful person subjectively assesses what is desired for the future to be probable or so important as to constrain belief and behaviour to be grounded upon its possibility (p. 227).

The intervention goal does not have to be immediate family rebuilding but rather stabilization of the family so the rebuilding process can begin when appropriate. Loss and bereavement adaptation is both a healing and rebuilding process, and a timetable cannot always be set (Kane, 1990).

The first meeting with the family, whether in the trauma center hospital, rehabilitation center, clinic, office, or family home, is vitally important. It sets the tone for the remaining family contacts. For example, if the initial family encounter is characterized by the health care professional's routine questions and a depersonalized explanation of brain injury, the remaining family counseling may be a procedural explanation, almost an intellectual exercise, not capturing, recognizing, or attending to the intense and profound emotions underlying the family's reaction to brain injury.

On the other hand, if, during the family visit, the health care professional assumes the role of a listener and a facilitator for the expression of feelings, and begins to comprehend, appreciate, and understand family dynamics, the remaining family visits and/or interventions will help the family members to understand their grief. Information at this point can be helpful if it is presented at a level that is congruent with individual family needs and relevant to their frame of reference. Sometimes too much information may not be helpful or relevant to the needs of the family at the time it is presented (Rolland, 1994).

During this first meeting and as family members attempt to experience and perhaps understand their own grief, good listening is shown by communicating a sense of caring, attending to the present family concerns, suspending judgements, and not attempting to compare the health care professional's experience with the family's experience unless it is helpful and relevant. This may be the case when the provider is a brain injury survivor or a family member, although this status alone does not guarantee a helpful or relevant perspective or intervention. Kane (1990) believes that effective helping with grief includes "maintaining a presence with the griever rather than solve the griever's problems ... not by attempting to remove the griever's pain, but instead, by allowing the griever to feel the pain of the loss" (p. 221). Walker and Pomeroy (1996) point out that caregivers who are grieving rather than depressed need support using the full range of their emotions toward the care recipient without the expectation that they will reach a stage of acceptance in some orderly predictable fashion.

Active listening can help the family because it communicates an acceptance of the family and invites the family members to share their worries and anxieties. Active listening also promotes the opportunity for family members to express themselves, namely, to express feelings and complaints without being judged. A response such as, "this is normal," is frequently the most reassuring information for the family. This is when the role of support groups can normalize the process and create a road map and benchmark for families (Appendix A).

At the initial family meetings, the health care provider should learn what the family understands about why the loss occurred, the effectiveness of the informal and formal supportive systems available to the family, and the family members' ability to cope effectively with stress. How an individual adapts after loss is generally determined by his or her individual coping skills. Matz (1978) has identified these goals as the determinants of successful grief resolution. The family must become aware of the basic source of the loss because what may be perceived by the health care professional as the cause of family grief may only be another symptom of a more serious problem. For example, the occurrence of a brain injury for a parent who has a long family history of alcoholism and absence from home for prolonged periods may renew feelings of resentment, especially if that person has undergone alcoholism rehabilitation before the diagnosis. Family members may still harbor deep emotions about the patient's earlier behavior. This represents unfinished business, and the new diagnosis aggravates these feelings because it symbolizes another source of unpleasantness for the family.

During family visits, it may be necessary for family members to review past events and repeat the events of the past, for this expression can help family members verbalize their feelings and then eventual make sense out of the loss. The family must ask the unanswerable "whys" over and over again before adjustment to the loss can take place. Piece by piece, the links with the past are re-examined, grieved, given up, and partially replaced with the hope that what is lost may be compensated for or even replaced by another source of personal or family satisfaction. While it may be important for families to ask "why," it may be more important for all involved to comprehend "why not."

As family members review the past and express their feelings about the loss in a non-judgmental context, as they begin to understand the implications of the loss to family life, they are making adaptive progress to a loss resolution. Adjustment to the loss involves change from the old ways at managing family responsibilities to a different outlook for the future, modifications in the family duties, and new choices for their own future.

Gradually, the family may adjust to the implications of the new situation resulting from the brain injury. The health care professional can often facilitate this change by sharing his or her own feelings in uncertain situations, engaging in relevant and personal disclosure, and challenging the family members to identify the advantages of making changes that result in loss adaptation. Family members should be active participants in the process as they search for new meaning and purpose while living with the brain injury trauma. This is not an easy task when living with the post-traumatic effect of a brain injury or other life losses.

When the health care professional has determined that the family members have a better understanding of the source of the loss, their reaction to it, and how adjustment could be achieved, and believes that a trusting relationship has been established with the family members, a course of action to meet the adjustment goals can be planned. The plan of action may take many forms, namely, providing support, reassurance, role models, information to help the family members move through the grief stages, and/or utilizing situational supports and resources. Grief resolution is encouraged by having a variety of well-integrated resources available to a family. Pastoral care, neighborhood crisis clinics, and friends can provide valuable assistance during the bereavement period. Identifying with others through support groups often helps toward both acceptance of the loss and acknowledgment that changes should be made in family life. Contact with the local chapter of the Brain Injury Association and other resources can be helpful (see Appendices A and B). While participation in these organizations and support groups is not a panacea to all of the issues and problems faced by a family, it provides the opportunity to learn from others who are in a similar place and can provide another dimension for social interaction.

The importance of social contacts is noted by Rosenthal et al. (1998) who point out that loss of friends and social contacts can last long after a brain injury. Families can learn from each other and be exposed to the common pitfalls of the recovery process.

The information imparted to a family should focus on more than the losses associated with brain injury. Although the loss may temporarily become the most striking feature of family life, the remaining resource opportunities should be emphasized. These resources are often the established family strengths or environmental supports readily available to family members. Providing information may frequently mean reinforcing health care knowledge, suggesting new expectations for the family members, or reviving expectations for each other that might have been lost at the onset of the brain injury. Through this information exchange process the health care professional assists the family members to both become aware of each other's needs and to learn how to use the networks of support both inside and outside the home.

The goal is to keep the family intact and to help members realize that "life can be worth living" during and after the brain injury experience. Rolland (1994) states: "A serious health crisis can awaken family members to opportunities for more satisfying, fulfilling relationships with each other. Hence any useful clinical model should emphasize the possibilities for growth, not just the liabilities and risks" (p. 10).

In looking toward the future and transcending grief, Davidhizar (1997) emphasizes that people with disabilities do not have to remain at the grief stage. Rather, "they can learn to accept their disabilities and adapt to symptoms while maintaining normalcy in their lives. Although their sources of satisfaction may change, their life satisfaction can be maintained" (p. 35). This is a key point because it places the trauma and loss in a context, focuses on the future life to live, and it is not limited by the life that was lost.

By supporting the learning of new information and skills while attending to each other's needs and expressing feelings, the family can begin the process of rebuilding, refocusing, and rejuvenating. However, this perspective is based upon the awareness that surviving and living beyond the trauma of a brain injury is hard work and that family members may not be able to progress at the same pace or reach their individual or common goals.

Throughout intervention, the family assumes the responsibility for any needed change. With the bereaved family there may be a terminating phase, but the members usually want the opportunity for periodic dialogue with the initial health care professional during the years that characterize adjustment to brain injury. They may want someone they can turn to when the painful reality of the loss occasionally becomes overwhelming. Consequently, contact with the family is important until it is mutually perceived that the family is coping successfully and does not need or desire further involvement with the health care professional. This is where self-help groups play a significant role because they are often more understanding and readily available to the person with brain injury and his or her family (see Appendix A).

Conclusion

The occurrence of a family loss related to brain injury is a powerful, encompassing, and dynamic experience. In order for family members to cope effectively they often need skillful and relevant intervention. This intervention must relate to the complexity of coping with a brain injury (Stoler and Hill 1998). Families need someone who can be there to listen, be a role model, offer reassurance, and provide and validate their feelings. For the family living with the reality of brain injury, intervention can take many forms but it is always guided by the conviction that underlying all approaches is the willingness to share another's loss as well as hopes and dreams. Such sharing is frequently the beginning of a resolution of the family loss and recognition that life is livable even though it will never be exactly the same. The power of perspective and hope is that it creates a vision for the future, clarifies the present, and contains the past. As one spouse poignantly stated, "Don't ever take away our hope for recovery" (Mulder, 1998).

The following personal statement, *For Better or For Worse*, by David Collins, explores the reality of living in spite of a brain injury and a spinal cord injury. It considers the complexities related to being a survivor, husband, father, and emerging person who is challenging the future and transcending the past.

Personal statement

For better or for worse
by David

Growing up in a family as the youngest of three boys, competition and survival were natural qualities. Athletics followed and played an important part of my life. During high school, my time was spent practicing for the upcoming game and "getting by" in the classroom to maintain eligibility. In college, my priorities changed and academics were goals I pursued to stay out of the draft more than anything else. At 23, Valerie, the girl I met in college, and I walked down the church aisle and professed our love to those in attendance. Nine months and three days later, we welcomed an addition to our union. As a coach and teacher, my skills were enhanced at classes or clinics; parenting, I hoped, would be a natural talent. As Kerry started to grow and reach her second birthday, we were good pals. If she misbehaved, this coach would make her sit on her plastic chair and not get up — probably a theory I had read about from one of my coaching journals. As Kerry grew, so did Valerie. She was expecting our second child in April. After some thinking, I chose to give up coaching and go into real estate sales and tax work. With a family it was important to look to the future and be prepared. I would make my mark and my family would enjoy the benefits. My planning was poor. After I played my last Christmas basketball game with fellow coaches, we convened at the local pub to review the game. After drinking beer and eating breakfast, I got in my car to drive home. Halfway home, I fell asleep and struck a utility pole while sitting atop my seatbelt. My life was instantaneously altered. As my pregnant wife entered the hospital emergency room at 4:00 a.m., the neurosurgeon blasted her about my high alcohol reading and poor prognosis. If I survived I'd need constant attention.

The accident occurred on December 27. My first recollection was in March. I called my wife by her maiden name, asked if we had any children, and displayed not only confusion, but an indifference as well. I was not only brain injured, but I was a quadriplegic. At one point, I was convinced they had wheeled my bed up a floor to the obstetrics section, and I vividly remembered delivering a baby. My days were spent going to therapy and returning to bed and watching television. A young man started visiting and sharing his story. His name was Dave and he had fallen out of a tree and broken his back 7 years earlier when he was 16 years old. He was very muscular as he wheeled around the halls and explained things like driving a car with hand controls, bowel and bladder control, and sexual activities with his dates. Dave got me out of my room and wheeling outside; he explained his life in graduate school to me and it was appealing. In time I chose to attend graduate school at the University of Illinois, renowned for its accessible campus and wheelchair sports programs. After 6 months in the hospital, I was allowed to go home for weekends. My expectations upon returning home were that my relationship with my daughter and my wife would be as they were before. My foremost thought was to resume sexual activity with Valerie and provide for both our needs. At 27, I had serious doubts about being a person or a man and felt the only way to prove my virility was in the bedroom. Valerie was very patient and empathic to my needs. My hygiene was terrible, a tracheostomy was done on my throat, my bladder and bowel needed to be emptied prior to commencing intimacy, and there was always the chance of having an accident. To this day, I will always be indebted to her for allowing me to believe "I was a man." I told her she gave Oscar winning performances when I needed them.

When I made it home permanently and re-entered the family unit, it had become apparent that Kerry, our precocious three year old, had taken my place. She had to be moved out of the king-size bed and back to her room. My adjustment to returning home, I had told Valerie, would be unnoticeable — or so I thought. My first morning home, I had forgotten to put my clothes next to my bed on the wheelchair (dressing is done prone on the bed). After 15 minutes of yelling for Valerie, I finally got, "Yeah what?" to which I requested she get my pants for me, which were on the floor. "I'm changing the baby and can't get back to you for 45 minutes," she said. I was livid. "Bullshit," I mumbled as I got in my chair, retrieved my trousers, and, getting back in bed, got dressed. Upon coming out to the kitchen and observing

Valerie drinking coffee and reading a magazine, I let loose. "What in the hell is going on?!" I screamed. After 5 minutes of ranting, I stormed off. Today, Valerie and I use this story at workshops and seminars on coping to health care professionals and families. We refer to this as the "Pants Story," and the lesson we convey is that never again did I forget my pants. I'm sure it was hard for Valerie to hear my pleas and not give in, but the lesson we learned is it is a disservice to perform a task for an individual without his or her attempting the feat first.

As time progressed, I entered graduate school and due to the insight of my counselor, who suggested that only two courses be taken to start out, I succeeded. As I wheeled across the street on a campus of 45,000 students, my name was yelled out and I stopped. A fellow approached and asked, "Didn't you play basketball for Brother Rice in Chicago?" "Yeah," I said, and as we continued our discussion, I recognized him as a wide receiver for a rival high school in Chicago. He went on to tell me he was pursuing his Ph.D. in therapeutic recreation/administration. He then asked if I would be interested in going out for the track team. The bewilderment on my face led him to explain therapeutic recreation and how the University of Illinois had wheelchair track, basketball, football, and a variety of other sports for those who are physically challenged. Practices were to start in two weeks. At my first practice, I was amazed to see the number of participants and their varying levels of function. I started to bring my daughter to practices and all of us seemed to enjoy ourselves. At various meets, my family would join me when ribbons were awarded and have their pictures taken — each of us was proud. The practices and the meets turned into family outings. Valerie coordinated things well by loading the car with the kids, a wheelchair, and me. I could sense my becoming less competitive with the girls.

As they became older, they became interested in playing sports. As a former coach, I had to use restraint as I cheered on from the sidelines at their t-ball games. One parent asked me if I would assist him in coaching the girls' basketball team which both our daughters were on. Reluctantly, I agreed, but again my daughters were proud of their dad sitting on the courtside bench. We truly began to communicate better and spoke about events that occured in the practices or games.

I followed both girls as they progressed through the years. When they were younger, they didn't know that fathers on wheelchairs weren't cool. As they grew older, their parents knew less than they did, but I could tell that had nothing to do with my being in a wheelchair — just a normal reaction to parents. One time, as I pulled into a mall, Kerry asked, "Why do you park in wheelchair parking?" "Why not?" I replied. "You compete in 10K races and can wheel better than some of these older people can walk," she said. I thought for a few minutes and felt somewhat flattered and responded, "Yeah, I suppose you're right." "It sounds like a special favor you're taking advantage of," she said. "I'll remember that in the future" was my response.

It was August when both girls asked if I would drive them and their friends to an amusement park. Our group had about eight people waiting in a long line to ride the attraction. As we sweltered in 90° temperature, a woman who took tickets came up to me and asked, "Are you familiar with our wheelchair policy?" I said no, and she explained that any wheelchair patrons and their guests do not have to wait in line. They may go to the front and stay on the ride for a second time if they chose. I looked at my oldest daughter and said, "I don't know. It kind of sounds like a special favor to me. What do you think?" "Oh no, dad. This is okay this time." Later in the month, my wife offered to take the girls to the same amusement park to which they quickly responded, "Can Dad come?"

In my relationships with my spouse and daughters, I live by showing them that we all have choices —sometimes because of our behavior we must accept the consequences. We all have special qualities and are unique. When we speak to others, communication is stressed as very important. Times are difficult for a lot of people and the key to my living is accepting and liking myself and taking it one day at a time.

During graduate school, I went to see the psychologist who worked at the rehabilitation center to inquire about what personal changes might I expect. His response stayed with me and makes a lot of sense: "If you were an S.O.B. before using a wheelchair, the chances are, post-trauma, you will be an S.O.B. in a wheelchair." The point is we usually don't plan bad things to happen to us: trauma, divorce, death, etc., but we still have the opportunity to change. Some are given a second chance, but that alone does not mean success. We are all individuals who need to work on our relationships within families as well as outside families. If we take one day at a time and keep a positive attitude, good things can result. In dealing with others, I clarify that my point is not to downplay or minimize trauma and its consequences. However, when one feels good about himself or herself, regardless of the circumstances he or she can share routine feelings with others. Each of us has a choice — choice can never be taken away.

Allied health providers and all members in society, must recognize each individual as unique and possessing skills others don't have. No two people are alike — uniqueness in abilities is our gift to one another.

Discussion questions on the personal statement

1. What is lost/gained when a young athlete is faced with changes subsequent to a disability? Are there any inherent or positive traits an athlete may possess to aid the process of rehabilitation?
2. How can long-term goals be a source of stress for a person whose life is altered by a brain injury? How does this compare with the immediate stress related to hygiene, dressing, eating, etc.?
3. Is a single person with a brain injury better off than a married person with young children? Is someone with a congenital disability better off than a person who experiences a mid-life trauma and must learn to adapt at age 50 to the demands of daily living?

4. How does the problematic relationship between alcohol and athletics manifest itself? Are roles of self-esteem and peer pressure relevant and contributory?
5. Was the response of the neurosurgeon helpful to David's wife?
6. How would you respond if your spouse did not remember who you were and whether or not you had children?
7. How can exposure to role models be a positive or stressful experience (e.g., having David meet with an active person who has mastered a disability)?
8. How can the need for intimacy become a major priority for a person returning home from the hospital? How did Valerie facilitate the adjustment? What if the roles were reversed and Valerie had the injury? What issues could emerge?
9. How could re-entry into the family have been facilitated by creative discharge planning?
10. How would your spouse respond if he or she had to choose between your needs and those of a child?
11. Why were sports a critical element in David's adjustment to his family?
12. What are the issues for children in adjusting to a parent with a brain injury? How is the age of a child a mitigating factor in the adjustment process?
13. What does David mean when he states, "Each of us has a choice?"
14. What would your challenges be if you were in David's situation?
15. How can a person or a family be proactive in the adjustment to a brain injury?
16. Discuss the role of hope.

Set 13. Why us?

Perspective

Most families live life hoping and expecting they will avoid the traumas and tragedies that are part of the life experience. No one can find fault with this perspective and hopefully most families will avoid the overwhelming traumas, tragedies, and losses that occur. However, when a trauma does occur it becomes an integral part of the family's life experience. In these situations, most families tend to focus their resources and make the necessary accommodations, often reaching a level of life functioning that is balanced and manageable. The vulnerability of most families in this situation is that they believe that nothing could be worse. Unfortunately, one trauma or brain injury does not make a person immune or insulated from additional loss and grief.

Loss, grief, and bereavement are part of the life and living process. Unfortunately, the losses and the subsequent grief are sad, painful, and distressing.

With a brain injury, the losses may be major, minor, or somewhere in between. Often the loss associated with a brain injury is magnified by prior losses and the unresolved pain associated with the loss experience.

Exploration

1. What was the most important thing you have lost in your life?
2. Who was the most important person you have lost?
3. What have you done or not done to help you resolve the loss and minimize the pain?
4. How has or how would a brain injury experience intensify prior losses?
5. What advice, help, or insights could you give a family member who cannot stop focusing on what he or she lost as a result of a brain injury?
6. How would you and your family feel and act if you sustained a TBI, recovered, and were diagnosed with multiple sclerosis?
7. How would you feel if you had a brain injury and your spouse decided to place you in a nursing home so that better care could be given to your child who had a chronic illness?
8. Identify and discuss how relationships with others have changed during your lifespan.
9. Were any of these changes a result of unresolved issues between family members related to illness, disability, or death?
10. What message has your family given to you regarding why people are injured?
11. What would be the first thing your family would say to you if you were head-injured because you were driving under the influence of alcohol?
12. How would your spouse respond if you refused to buy a bicycle helmet for your child and as a result the child sustained a brain injury?

References

Bowlby, J. (1980) *Attachment and Loss: Loss, Sadness and Depression*, Vol. 3, Basic Books, New York.

Brown, J.C. (1990) Loss and grief: an overview and guided imagery intervention model, *J. of Ment. Health Counseling*, 12(4), 434–445.

Brown, T.J. and Stoudemine, A.G. (1983) Normal and pathological grief, *J. of the Am. Med. Assoc.*, 250, 378–382.

Bugen, L.A. (1977) Human grief: a model for prediction and intervention, *Am. J. of Orthopsychiatr.*, 47, 196–206.

Davidhizar, R. (1997) Disability does not have to be the grief that never ends: helping patients adjust, *Rehabil. Nursing*, 22(1), 32–35.

DeBoskey, D.S. (1996) *Coming Home: A Discharge Manual for Families of Persons with Brain Injury*, HDI, Houston.

Doka, K.J. (1995) Children Mourning, Mourning Children, Hospice Foundation of America, Washington, D.C.

Fell, M. (1994) Helping older children grieve: a group therapy approach, *Health Visitor*, 67(3), 92–94.

Gallagher, D., Rose, J., Rivera, P., Lovett, S., and Thompson, L.W. (1989) Prevelance of depression in families care givers, *Gerontol.*, 29, 449–456.

Gardner, D. (1999) The "Protective Barrier" in Brain Injury, TBI Challenge, Brain Injury Association, April/May, 3(2), 8.

Garner, J. (1997) Dementia: an intimate death, *Br. J. of Med. Psychol.*, 70(2), 177–184.

Gilewski, M.J and Zelinski, E.M. (1995) Loss and grief, in *The Encyclopedia of Disability and Rehabilitation*, Dell Orto, A.E. and Marinelli, R.P., Eds., Simon & Schuster/Macmillan, New York.

Gomez-Hernandez, R., Max, J., Kosier, T., Paradiso, S., Robinson, R. (1997) Social impairment and depression after traumatic brain injury, *Arch. of Phys. Med. And Rehabil.*, 78, 1321–1326.

Heiney, S., Hasan, L., and Price, K. (1993) Developing and implementing a bereavement program for a children's hospital, *J. of Pediatr. Nursing*, 8(6), 385–391.

Kane, B. (1990) Grief and the adaptation to loss, *Rehabil. Educ.*, 4, 213–224.

Kapust, L.R. and Weintraub, S. (1984) Living with a family member suffering from Alzheimer's Disease, in *Helping Patients and Their Families Cope with Medical Problems*, Roback, H.D., Ed., Josey-Bass, San Francisco, p. 462.

Kubler-Ross, E. (1983) On Children and Death, Macmillan, New York.

Matz, M. (1978) Helping families cope with grief, in *Helping Clients with Special Concerns*, Eisenberg, S. and Patterson, L., Eds., Rand McNally College, Chicago, 218–238.

McKinlay, W. and Hickox, A. (1988) How can families help in the rehabilitation of the head injured?, *J. of Head Trauma Rehabil.*, 3(4), 64–72.

Miles, M.S. and Crandell, E.K. (1983) The search for meaning and its potential for affecting growth in bereaved parents, *Health Values*, Achieving High Level Wellness, 7(1), 19–23.

Milligan, S.E., Ed. (1984) *Community Health Care for Chronic Physical Illness: Issues and Models*, Case Western Reserve University, Cleveland, 44–48.

Miller, T.W., Houston, L., and Goodman, R. (1994) Clinical issues in psychosocial rehabilitation for spouses with physical disabilities, *J. of Dev. and Phys. Disabil.*, 6(1), 50.

Moldonado, J.L., Fernandez, F., Garza-Trevino, E., and Levy, J. (1997) Depression and its treatment in neurological disease, *Psychiatr. Ann.*, 27(5), 341–346.

Mulder, P. (1998) Proceeding 17, TBI Challenge symposium, Brain Injury Association, Dec., 2, 9.

Nunn, K. (1996) Personal hopefulness: a conceptual review of the relevance of the perceived future to psychiatry, *Br. J. of Med. Psychol.*, 69, 227–245.

Parkes, C.M. (1972) *Bereavement: Studies of Grief in Adult Life*, Tavistock, London.

Parkes, C.M. (1975) Determinants of outcome following bereavement, *Omega*, 6, 303–323.

Parkes, C.M. (1985) Bereavement, *Br. J. of Psychiatr.*, 146, 11–17.

Pollock, G.H. (1961) Mourning and adaptation, *Int. J. of Psychoanal.*, 42, 341–361.

Rando, T.A. (1986) A comprehensive analysis of anticipatory grief: perspectives, processes, promises, and problems, in *Loss and Anticipatory Grief*, Rando, T.A., Ed., Lexington Books, Lexington, MA.

Reichley, M. (1995) Patients and caregivers cope with grief in rehabilitation, *Adv. for Speech-Language Pathol.*, 5(19), 18.

Rocchio, C. (1998) Family News and Views, Brain Injury Association, Oct. 2.

Rolland, J.S. (1994) *Families, Illness and Disabilty: An Integrative Treatment Model*, Basic Books, New York.

Rosenthal, M., Christensen, B., and Ross, T. (1998) Depression following traumatic brain injury, *Arch. of Phys. Med. and Rehabil.*, Jan, 79, 90–103.

Silverman, P. (1981) *Helping Women Cope with Grief*, Sage, Beverly Hills, CA.

Stoler, D.R. and Hill, B.A. (1998) *Coping with Mild Traumatic Brain Injury*, Avery Publishing Group, Garden City, NY.

Stroebe, M., Gergen, M., Gergen, K., and Stroebe, W. (1992) Broken hearts or broken bonds: Love and death in historical perspective, *Am. Psychol.*, 47(10), 1205–1212.

Walker, R.J. and Pomeroy, E.C. (1996) Depression or Grief? The experience of caregivers of people with dementia, *Health and Soc. Work*, 21(4), 247–254.

Wright, H. and Oliver, G. (1993) *Kids Have Feelings Too*, Victor Books, Chicago.

Zemzars, I.S. (1984) Adjustment to health loss: implications for psychosocial treatment, in *Community Health Care For Chronic Physical Illness: Issues and Models*, Milligan, S.E., Ed., Case Western Reserve University, Cleveland, OH, 44–48.

Zisook, S. and DeVaul, R. (1985) Unresolved grief, *Am. J. of Psychoanal.*, 45(4), 370–379.

chapter ten

Alcohol and disability: a brain injury perspective

Perspective

Alcohol use and abuse will always guarantee that people will be acquiring brain injuries, complicating already precarious situations, resulting in families who will be faced with a lifetime of caregiving, misery, and increased distress. It is quite a legacy, which somehow is not reflected in alcohol advertisements that promise bliss yet deliver misery. Alcohol abuse is often a one-way ticket to brain injury trauma, treatment, and rehabilitation.

This chapter will explore the issues related to alcohol and disability in general, relating them to brain injury and placing them in a treatment and rehabilitation context. Whether we drink or not, everyone is a potential consumer of the toxic consequences related to alcohol, and we are all potential victims.

Concern about alcohol was expressed more than 100 years ago by Blair (1888). He wrote:

> The conflict between man and alcohol is as old as civilization, more destructive than any other form of warfare, and as fierce to-day [sic] as at any time since the beginning.
>
> It is not an exaggeration to say that no other evil known in human history has been of such vast proportions and lamentable consequences as that of alcoholic intemperance. As the whole past of the race has been cursed by it, so its whole future is threatened with increasing calamity, unless there be a period put to its ravages.
>
> It is a peculiarity of this curse that it is developed by civilization, and then, like the parricide, it destroys the source of its own life.

> But although alcohol is his special foe, it by no means confines its dagger and chalice to civilized man. Combining with the spirit of a mercenary commerce, this active essence of evil is hunting and extirpating the weaker races and indigenous populations of uncivilized countries from the face of the earth (p. ix).

These timeless thoughts reflect several issues which are central in a discussion of alcohol and its relation to disability in general and brain injury in particular.

The common themes are:

- There is a war going on that has more victims than most conflicts of recent memory.
- The ravages of alcohol-induced illness, disability, and brain injury are complex, long-lasting, and often irreversible.
- The forces of alcohol's wrath and destruction are often driven by profit and commercial interests at the expense of the common good.
- Certain people are more vulnerable to the life-enhancing promises of alcohol-related advertising due to their pre-trauma or post-trauma cognitive, physical, and emotional limitations, but everyone is a potential victim.
- Treatment and rehabilitation efforts can be compromised by the presence of alcohol and other drugs.
- Alcohol may be used as a means of "normalization" and control when in fact it reduces control and increases the risk for "denormalization."

Alcohol abuse often causes a variety of problems for individuals, families, and society (Abel and Ziendenberg, 1985; Anda et al., 1988; Bratter and Forrest, 1985; Fallon, 1990; Harrison-Felix et al., 1998; Hingson and Howland, 1987; Huth et al., 1983; Jaffe et al., 1996; Jones, 1989; Kinney and Leaton, 1987; Kreutzer et al., 1990; Lehman et al., 1994; Lowenstein et al., 1990; Maio et al., 1997; Murphy et al., 1992; Noble, 1978; Schuckit, 1986, 1995a, 1995b, 1996; Shipley et al., 1990; Soderstrom and Cowley, 1987; Teplin et al., 1989; Waller, 1990; Waller et al., 1997; Yates et al., 1987; Zink et al., 1996).

Alcohol and disability

While there has been an increased awareness of the problems related to substance abuse by persons living with illness and disability, alcohol is still a cause of disability and a major impediment in treatment and rehabilitation (Beck et al., 1991; Benshoff and Leal, 1990; Boros, 1989; Cherry, 1988; Dean et al., 1985; Frieden, 1990; Greer, 1986; Greer and Walls, 1997; Heinemann et al., 1988; Heinemann et al., 1989; Heinemann, 1993; Krause, 1992; Kolakowsky-Hayner et al., 1999; Kirubakaran et al., 1986; Li and Ford, 1998; Lowenstein et al., 1990; Moore and Seigel, 1989; Moore et al., 1994; Moore and Ford, 1996; Moore and Li, 1998; Pires, 1989; Rasmussen and DeBoer, 1981; Rohe and Depompolo, 1985; Straussman, 1985; Tate, 1993; Waller, 1990; Wolkstein and Moore, 1996; Woosley, 1981).

It is clear that alcohol is an ongoing problem for those engaged in the treatment, rehabilitation, and caregiving of persons living with the illnesses and disabilities related to "fall out" from alcohol abuse.

Dual diagnosis

Families and individuals are faced with the often complex and demanding consequences of brain injury, but there is an added stress when alcohol and substance abuse result in a multi-dimensional disability and present a unique set of problems related to dual diagnosis.

The long-term consequences of and limited treatment resources for brain-injured substance abusers is discussed by Sparadeo et al. (1990):

> It is becoming more common to see addicted or severe-
> ly troubled substance abusers several years after a
> brain injury. These individuals are usually referred to
> a postacute brain injury rehabilitation facility or a sub-
> stance abuse program. Unfortunately, treatment op-
> portunities for these dual diagnosis cases are very
> limited (p. 4).

The importance and complexity of dual diagnosis related to mental illness and substance abuse is stated in the literature (Doyle-Pita, 1995; Carey, 1989; Daley et al., 1987; Drake et al., 1998; Greenbaum et al., 1996; Kofoed et al., 1986; Kofoed and Keys, 1998; McKelvy et al., 1987; Minkoff and Ajilore, 1998; Mueser and Fox, 1998; Brown et al., 1989; Sciacca and Thompson, 1996; Sternberg, 1986).

The challenging reality for families of persons who are mentally ill is that they are often overwhelmed by the demands and problems associated with the primary diagnosis of mental illness. Consequently, they may not be concerned about, aware of, or able to cope with the potential problems associated with the synergistic effects of mental illness and alcohol abuse which could result in another physical disability such as brain injury. In an opposite situation, a person with traumatic brain injury (TBI) is at risk for a secondary disability such as a psychiatric disability.

Hibbard et al. (1998) state that TBI is a risk factor for psychiatric disabil-ities, and they expressed concern related to substance abuse disorders post TBI:

> Psychiatric disorders are frequent sequelae of trau-
> matic brain injury. Long term residual psychiatric se-
> quelae pose challenges to community reentry and to
> quality of life and are often viewed as more seriously

handicapping than the cognitive and physical sequelae of the injury itself (p. 24).

The potential for this is clarified when suicide attempts are related to
mental illness complicated by substance abuse. It is important to realize that
if a suicide attempt is not successful, there may still be irreversible physical
and emotional consequences for the patient and the family.

An example of this is poignantly illustrated using a case of a young man
who had a history of mental illness and alcohol abuse. He attempted suicide
by jumping from a building. He survived with a severe brain injury complicated by a spinal cord injury. This was an overwhelming tragedy for the
family who had successfully focussed on and adjusted to the long-term
demands of psychiatric disorder and a substance abuse problem; they were
not prepared for the additional demands of TBI complicated by quadriplegia.
This situation can be best captured by a statement made by his parent:

> One lesson we have learned is that we never say it
> cannot get worse. It certainly can but that also creates
> the possibility that things can also get better. In living
> with a brain injury we certainly have experienced both.
> Now we are prepared for the worse, expect the best,
> and try to make it happen. If not, at least we were
> aware and not kidding ourselves.

When disability is conceptualized as a loss of control over one's physical
or emotional destiny, the stage is then set for some to cope with the concomitant stress, pain, grief, and depression by initiating or increasing their use
of and dependency on alcohol and other drugs (Frisbie and Tun, 1984;
Woosley, 1981).

The irony of the substance abuse process is that even though it has
resulted in a severe disability, some individuals may still rely on drugs and
alcohol to cope with their physical and emotional losses (Greer, 1986; Greer
et al., 1990). However, it is important to consider that among persons living
with disabilities there are those who had a problem with substance abuse
prior to the disability, as well as those persons who began using alcohol or
other drugs following the onset of a disability.

The problem for many individuals and families challenged by alcohol is
intensified when they realize that forces in our society have the power to
impair, maim, and kill their children, friends, strangers, spouses, parents, and
themselves. A direct result of this reality is the pervasive helplessness most
people feel in controlling their destiny and the wellbeing of their loved ones.

Violence related to alcohol often results in difficult emotional and physical situations. Shapiro (1982) discussed the relationship between alcohol and
family violence and indicated that family members are often the direct victims of violence resulting in trauma and disability. In addition to acts of
physical abuse such as wife battering or shaken baby syndrome, there are

often long-term and irreversible consequences, such as brain injury, which may be a direct or indirect consequence of alcohol-induced violence caused by strangers or even family members. Unfortunately, when family members are the cause of the problem and the loss, these situations often result in unforgettable realities that can be more consuming to the family than the forgiving, understanding successful rehabilitation of the abusing family member who caused the brain injury of a loved one, even if it was by default rather than intent.

An additional consideration in a discussion of alcohol and its relationship to disability and brain injury is how a family uses or abuses alcohol. If a family's alcohol use is casual, there may be a negative reaction when the effects of alcohol abuse by a family member conflict with familial value systems and traditions. Frequently alcohol use is condoned by the family because it is considered recreational and less harmful than illegal drugs. This tolerant position can change dramatically if under the influence of alcohol, a loved one is involved in a vehicular accident and becomes disabled or brain injured. It is within this transition from alcohol use to irreparable harm that most families find their ultimate agony, pain, and regret.

Alcohol use and abuse will create personal and familial stress because illness, disability, and brain injury are direct and indirect consequences. When discussing alcohol, one must keep in mind that alcohol is a drug, as Fort (1973) stated more than a quarter of a century ago:

> … alcohol is our most widely used mind-altering drug.
> It is by far our hardest drug and constitutes our biggest
> drug problem in that it kills, disables, addicts, and
> makes psychotic more people than all the other drugs
> put together (p. v–vi).

In effect, not much has changed since 1973 except there is more denial of the problem, a distorted perception of the causes, and a lack of awareness of the real consequences, one of which is brain injury and all it represents, promises, and takes away from the person and the family.

Alcohol and brain injury

Faced with a reality that has been difficult to ignore, the field of brain injury rehabilitation has given serious attention to alcohol and its relation to brain injury. In a very powerful article, Kreutzer et al. (1990) articulate the relationship between alcohol and brain injury when they write, "Evidence clearly indicates there are interrelationships between alcohol use, risk for brain injury, and post-injury psychosocial adjustment." (p. 14).

A similar point is made by Seaton and David (1990):

> For the individual with TBI, substance abuse has a
> profoundly destructive influence. There is an increase

not only in the risk of reinjury, but also in the aggra-
vation of cognitive deficits and poor impulse control,
and a diminution of social skills (p. 44).

These themes and points have been articulated by an army of authors
and researchers who have further explored the multi-dimensional relationship between brain injury and alcohol (Alterman and Tarter, 1985; Corrigan
et al., 1999; Bonger et al., 1997; Bombardier et al., 1997; Bombardier et al.,
1997; Blackerby and Baumgarten, 1990; Bond, 1986; Burke et al., 1988, 1991;
Corrigan, 1995, 1996; Corrigan et al., 1995; Delmonico, Hanley-Peterson, and
Englander, 1998; Dikmen et al., 1995; Hibbard et al., 1998; Jones, 1989;
Kreutzer et al., 1990; Kreutzer et al., 1991; Kreutzer and Harris, 1990;
Kreutzer et al., 1996; Kreutzer et al., 1997; Kreutzer and Sander, 1997; Langley
and Kiley, 1992; Miller, 1989; Ohio Valley Center for Brain Injury Prevention
and Rehabilitation, 1998; Peterson et al., 1990; Rimel et al., 1981; Rimel et
al., 1982; Rimel, 1982; Ruff et al., 1990; Ryan and Butters, 1983; Sander et al.,
1997; Sander et al., 1997; Solomon and Sparadeo, 1992; Sparadeo and Gill,
1989; Sparadeo et al., 1990; Sparadeo et al., 1992; Tobis et al., 1982; Zasler,
1991).

The complexity of the problem and the synergistic relationship between
alcohol and TBI are summarized by Langley (1991) in a literature review
related to the causal role of alcohol in the acquisition of TBI as well as its
deleterious effect on rehabilitation. Langley concludes:

- Alcohol use is involved in the acquisition of 35 to 66% of all traumatic
  brain injuries.
- Alcohol is also a key factor in the failure of community reintegration
  efforts for many clients.
- Alcohol detrimentally affects functions associated with the prefrontal
  and temporal lobes including memory, planning, verbal fluency, complex motor control, and the modulation of emotionality.
- Alcohol use may further reduce the capacity for behavioral self-regulation for clients who have compromised prefrontal-temporal functioning due to traumatic brain injury.

These observations present a complex and demanding reality for persons
and families who must adjust to initial losses related to alcohol use and live
with its ongoing and evolving consequences.

In discussing why brain injury survivors turn to alcohol, Sparadeo et al.
(1990) state:

> Brain injury survivors are particularly vulnerable to
> use of alcohol or other substances during or after the
> rehabilitation process, for several reasons. They must
> deal with the losses experienced following the injury.
> They are often alienated by their peers and treated

differently by family members. Activity levels are often curtailed, and a significant degree of boredom is a common experience. This combination of factors contributes greatly to the use of substances, particularly alcohol (p. 3).

The implications of alcohol abuse are clearly stated in the following:

Alcohol abuse has been associated with TBI in approximately half of all occurrences. Whether the TBI is a direct result of alcohol or other substance use, or if it predates the substance abuse disability, the continued abuse of alcohol and other drugs can negate attempts at physical, social, and cognitive rehabilitation (SARDI, 1996).

A recent issue of *Brain Injury Rehabilitation Update* (1998) focuses on the importance of these issues:

It is no secret that alcohol abuse and traumatic injuries often go together, and brain injury is no exception ... those who do resume drinking may be compounding their problems rather than simply adding to them. The use of alcohol — even in a normal amount — is associated with poor neurological outcomes ... (p. 1).

Bogner and Lamb-Hart (1995) list the following eight points related to brain injury and alcohol and substance abuse:

1. People who use alcohol or other drugs after they have had brain injuries don't recover as much or as quickly as people who don't use alcohol or other drugs.
2. Brain injuries cause problems in balance, walking or talking that get worse when a person uses alcohol or other drugs.
3. People who have had brain injuries often say or do things without thinking first, a problem that is made worse by using alcohol or other drugs.
4. Brain injuries cause problems in thinking, like concentration or memory, and using alcohol and other drugs makes these worse.
5. After a brain injury, alcohol and other drugs have a more powerful effect.
6. People who have had brain injuries are more likely to have times when they feel low or depressed and drinking alcohol and getting high on other drugs makes this worse.
7. After a brain injury, drinking alcohol or using other drugs can cause a seizure.

8. People who drink alcohol or use other drugs after brain injuries are more likely to have further brain injuries (p. 14).

Situational variables

When discussing disability, brain injury, and alcohol use, it is important to consider the many situational variables that can complicate the emotional rehabilitation process for the family. For example:

- Was the injured person an alcohol or substance abuser prior to the accident?
- Did alcohol have a role in the situation?
- Was the injured person in control or a victim (e.g., driver or passenger)?
- Was the person a non-substance user who was a victim of a drunk-driving situation? A crime of violence?
- Prior to the trauma, was alcohol part of the family's lifestyle?
- Did the person already have a brain injury which was then complicated by a subsequent injury related to alcohol?
- Are alcohol and other drugs threats to treatment and rehabilitation due to resumption of use or initiation of dependency?

While the drug or alcohol has had a major impact on a person's and family life, it does not mean that the problem has been understood, managed, or eliminated. This point is illustrated by the fact that some people who have sustained an alcohol-related brain injury or spinal cord injury may still drink and/or drink and drive and continue to place themselves and their families at risk.

The importance of this point is that there are stresses and residuals consequent to alcohol abuse which can be far more problematic than the alcohol abuse alone. The following case synopsis further illustrates this point:

> A person was referred for treatment with the presenting problem of adjusting to his brain injury. During the initial evaluation, a complex familial situation emerged. Prior to his injury, the individual was engaged in a problematic marital situation which involved alcohol abuse. The day the couple decided to obtain a divorce, the husband, while intoxicated, was severely head injured as a result of an industrial accident. He was hit by a truck and was comatose for 3 months. After a year of hospitalization and rehabilitation, he still had major cognitive difficulties and physical limitations. During this time his wife did not visit and wanted to get on with the divorce and on with her life. The harsh reality was that the complexity of the situation and financial considerations forced the cou-

ple to live together in a toxic environment clouded by anger, bitterness, and resentment. Just as alcohol was part of the pre-injury lifestyle, it became more of a problem during rehabilitation. This was manifested in physical and emotional abuse that culminated in legal action of charges of mutual assault and physical injury to the wife resulting in a complex physical, emotional, and legal situation.

Another case synopsis which illustrates the compounding nature of the effects of alcohol abuse is as follows:

A young woman sought out treatment for the presenting problem of chronic alcohol abuse and concern about her marriage. During treatment, her husband expressed his intentions to file for a divorce. When this occurred, the client, while under the influence of alcohol, went out for a drive and crashed into a tree. She sustained severe head trauma, was facially disfigured, and lost an arm as well as sight in one eye. In addition, she needed many surgical procedures related to her broken hips and legs. Her husband promised not to seek the divorce if she would sign all of their assets over to him. When this occurred, he left the country, leaving her destitute and suicidal. When asked about his actions he stated that he did not want to be married to a cripple. Her response was to drink heavily, placing her physical and emotional health in jeopardy and necessitating intensive alcohol treatment and rehabilitation.

Both these case summaries reflect the enormity and complexity of the disability experience for couples who are stressed by a physical and emotional realities complicated by alcohol use. In both cases, the marital system was problematic prior to the brain injury and collapsed when the added stress of the brain injury experience took an additional toll. However, it must be pointed out that there are occasions when a dysfunctional marital or familial system can improve if it can respond to the challenges of a disability by initiating new behaviors and establishing more functional roles. This occurred in the following case synopsis:

A young couple who had been married for 5 years were on the verge of a separation. This situation was a result of several years of individual alcohol abuse and domestic violence. The result was that the couple lived in the same house but led very separate lives. They had two children whom they both cared for. One evening

the young woman was in an alcohol-related accident
which was life-threatening and was complicated by a
brain injury. Her husband responded to the crisis by
stopping his drinking, organizing the family, and
working toward the wellbeing and rehabilitation of his
wife. A year later, they both were alcohol-free, intact
as a family, and were appreciative of the gains that were
a direct result of trauma and loss. The young man said
it best when he stated, "I guess our lives were so out
of control and distorted by alcohol that we both needed
something serious to happen to get our attention."

For some families, their lives are complicated by the reality that they
must be vigilant in their efforts to eliminate the disastrous consequences of
alcohol while often being forced into roles and situations that are complicated at best. The challenge is not only to cope with a brain injury but also
to live with the losses related to poor choices and often irreversible consequences. This situation is further complicated by the fact that at any time
during the lifespan, families can be forced into caregiver, supportive, or
custodial roles that they find stressful, demanding, and frustrating. In
attempting to negotiate this complex process, families are often faced with
the reality of their loss and the limitation of their resources. As a result, the
nuclear family may feel powerless. Contributing to this powerlessness is the
media which has created norms slanted toward the hedonistic lifestyle made
attainable by alcohol use. On a daily basis, children, adolescents, and adults
are bombarded by advertisements which create the image that alcohol is a
vehicle to self-fulfillment, enjoyment, and excitement when in reality it is a
potential shortcut to brain injury, trauma, chaos, coma management, death,
and familial collapse. This point is made by Miller (1989) when he states:

> One need hardly comment on the glorification of life
> in the fast lane that deluges us in this country through
> advertising and the media, for example, TV beer com-
> mercials. No surprise, then, that impulsivity, drinking,
> driving and brain injury all go together so frequently
> in the United States, as well as elsewhere (p. 28).

When discussing problems related to aggressive behavior following
brain injury, Miller (1990) points out:

> The situation may be further compounded by the high
> rate of alcohol and drug abuse typically found in this
> group — substance abuse acting both as a causal factor
> in the injury itself (e.g., auto and industrial accidents),
> and as a postconcussion complication in lowering the

seizure threshold or further exacerbating disinhibition in a frontally-compromised individual (p. 16).

Conclusion

The destructive power of alcohol abuse is a realistic threat which may consume its victims and create a state of loss, failure, and helplessness. A person may die, be psychologically fragmented, be imprisoned by a brain injury, and be the cause of a variety of personal and familial tragedies. In attempting to control these realities, families are faced with the task of self-examination, self-exploration, and often self-incrimination as they attempt to define their roles as either part of the problem or the solution.

The challenge of working with persons and families living with a brain-injured member and the ongoing threats and consequences of alcohol abuse, is mobilizing those resources and supports which can be stabilizing factors during an ongoing rehabilitation process.

To focus on the future benefits of treatment and rehabilitation without the development of viable alternatives to alcohol and other forms of substance abuse, is ignoring the potential vulnerability of the population and the potential role of alcohol in a person's life. This is a significant issue because an individual who makes a commitment to treatment and rehabilitation often assumes that there is a chance to survive and attain a reasonable quality of life. If the skills cannot be utilized in the real world, relapse becomes a reality and those responsible for the design and expectations of the brain injury treatment and rehabilitation process must bear the burden of failure and not project blame onto their clients. This point is particularly relevant for the person with a brain injury who must continue to meet the challenges of the life and living process without alcohol use and its concomitant pathology and often irreversible consequences. As Langley (1991) states:

> For TBI clients, however, an accurate appraisal of the harmfulness of drinking may be difficult due to damage to those areas of the brain which subtend perception and understanding. The client seems unable to call to mind any negative consequences. Positive expectancies for the benefits of alcohol are often more resilient, and in the face of failure to cope with high-risk situations, could reduce motivation to abstain (p. 256).

While there are many important issues related to the treatment and rehabilitation of persons living with brain injuries, there are also important issues related to the role of alcohol as a cause of illness, disability, brain injury, loss, and death. How can we be content as a society who reacts to the problems consequent to alcohol use but ignores the facts and minimizes the reality? Until we acknowledge and respond to the pervasive and causal role alcohol plays in the creation of illness, disability, and brain injury, we are doomed to be victims of a double standard that decries the by-products of alcohol abuse but revels in the media distortion which presents people with a dream and delivers a nightmare. Alcohol, in effect, is the "Trojan horse" of the brain injury treatment and rehabilitation process.

The following personal statement, *Attitude is Everything, A Father's Perspective* poignantly illustrates the life-altering reality when drinking and driving result in brain damage, loss, and ongoing emotional trauma which are made bearable by having reasonable goals and a positive attitude.

Personal statement

Attitude is everything, a father's perspective

Life sure deals some unexpected cards. I was convinced that I had gotten through the rough times in my life. After I married my second wife, life seemed almost perfect. She and her two boys and my son and I were becoming a happy family until the day that tragedy struck us. A woman who had been to a retirement party where she drank too much, got behind the wheel of a car, plowed into my son, and almost killed him. The doctors in the trauma center said he would live but that we should start looking for nursing homes because his brain damage would cause him to be a vegetable. Why do they say things like that? I figure because they don't really know but they want to prepare you for the worst so you won't be shocked. When I think about it, I still get mad. It's a good thing that we didn't listen to them.

My first wife and I had my son when I was 21 so when he had his accident 2 years ago when he was 19, I was only 40, and my second wife was 35. Her boys were younger, of course, but we were definitely out of the babysitting stage. We were still young and free to do what we wanted without having to worry about the kids all the time.

After the accident, all that changed. We had a "child" who needed to be watched constantly at first. After a while, we tested him to see if we could leave him alone for longer periods of time. It wasn't a big problem because we're a family that has always done things together, so on the weekends we all worked on the house that we're now building on our property in Pennsylvania. During the week we had the most difficulty because both my wife and I work; she's a bank manager and I'm a mason. In the beginning, different people from our church would come and stay with my son. After a while, they needed to be there less and less. We're believers in the power of positive thinking. If you believe that someone can eventually be independent even when he's brain injured, you'll pass that optimistic attitude onto him. My wife was an independent child while growing up and she wouldn't let him act helpless. She kept expecting my son to take more and more responsibility. It was a little rough for her because at times she felt guilty about being hard on him, especially when the progress was slow. She went to talk to a counselor about it. The counselor helped her see that she couldn't fix him — that he would have to fix himself — that but it was okay to have expectations that eventually he would be more responsible. My wife's a backbone for this family. Sometimes I get real impatient if things move too slowly, but she convinces me that in time things will work out if we work at it. I know she's right. Even though my son's in a wheelchair most of the time, he can now stay alone, pickup the house, and a couple of times a week, he makes dinner. The good news is he's going back to school to learn about computers. Before the accident, he had no ambition to have a career. All he cared about was girls and sports. He definitely was not a great student. Now he still is not a great student, but he does have ambition. We know that it will be slow going. One thing about head-injured people is that even if they intend to do things, they can be very slow while doing them. One minute it seems he's forgotten what he said he was going to do. That's improving because he knows that he has to do his homework or he'll be embarrassed when he goes to class. It's good because he gets to be around other people and he needs that. If you were to ask him what's the hardest thing about life after the injury, he'd say not being able to walk, but if you ask me I'd say not having a normal social life. He wants a girlfriend in the worst way and was very depressed for a long time because he thought he'd never have one. Before the accident, he was a leader type, sure of himself and he had lots of friends and girlfriends. Now, because he talks slowly and so softly, he's very self-conscious, and for a long time he avoided people his own age. When he was in the rehabilitation center, he met girls who were head-injured also, but I know he really wants to meet a "normal" girl. As my wife says, "He was sweet before the accident and he's still that way and eventually he'll find someone who appreciates him."

I'm convinced the Lord works in strange ways. Since the accident, we're even closer as a family. The younger boys help their older brother. Of course, they fight like brothers, too, but they've learned compassion. We try hard not to neglect them because of their older brother's needs; we know if we did, they'd resent him and we don't want that to happen. We haven't given up our dreams — just reorganized them. My wife was going to go to college full-time, and now she'll go part-time. We were going to build our house in 5 years, and now we'll take 10 years to build. It's been interesting to design a house that could accommodate a person in a wheelchair. Even if my son leaves home and lives on his own, he'll always have a comfortable home to visit. If you want something and you're willing to work hard for it, you'll get it some way. Attitude is everything.

Discussion questions on the personal statement

1. How does surviving crises and making a new beginning create emotional vulnerability?
2. What is an adequate sentence for a person who kills someone in a drunk-driving accident? Who causes an accident that results in a brain injury?

3. Do you think that the suggestion made by the doctors in the trauma center that the father should start looking for a nursing home because his son would be a vegetable was helpful? Why or why not?
4. Discuss the impact of a brain injury when it occurs at various stages of childrearing.
5. Develop a respite care program that would respond to the unique needs of this family.
6. How can the power of positive thinking be an asset, as well as a liability?
7. Discuss the positive and negative implications of the statement, "My wife was an independent child while growing up and she wouldn't let him act helpless."
8. How can a brain injury result in new career goals and ambition for academic as well as vocational goals?
9. Give examples of how a person with a brain injury can perceive loss differently from parents or significant others.
10. Should individuals with brain injuries be encouraged to date or marry people with brain injuries?
11. How can a brain injury experience make a family closer?
12. What is meant by the statement, "We haven't given up our dreams — just reorganized them?"
13. Give examples of how the concept of working hard to attain a goal can provide hope as well as frustration.
14. Should the makers and sellers of alcohol be liable for producing a dangerous product?

Set 14. One for the road

Perspective

Since many brain injuries result from vehicular accidents, it seems reasonable to focus on the cause of the problem as well as the effects.

One consideration is that advertising often presents alcohol use as an integral part of daily life which includes recreation, socialization, and work.

Exploration

In order to better understand the scope of the issue, do the following:

1. Go through a variety of magazines and select alcohol advertisements that you think create distorted images.
2. Identify what groups of people you think would be most vulnerable.
3. Discuss the concept of potential consequences.
4. Explore how potential consequences could be presented in the media (e.g., "This wheelchair's for you.").

5. Should advertisers, brewers, and distillers be responsible for medical costs associated with brain injury consequent to drunk driving?
6. Should people with brain injuries be prevented from buying alcohol? Why or why not?
7. What disabilities are caused by alcohol?
8. What disabilities do you think could cause alcohol abuse?
9. How would you approach a person who said, "I lost so much as a result of my brain injury that I need to drink just to get by?"
10. If you were brain injured, would you tend to use or abuse alcohol? What factors would influence your decision?
11. Have you ever worked with a client whose substance abuse undermined the treatment and rehabilitation process?
12. Should the media be limited in the kind of alcohol advertising they present to the public?
13. If you were a judge presiding over a case in which a drunk driver killed a 17 year old and injured another 17 year old who survived brain injury, what do you think would be an appropriate sentence? What would be adequate compensation for each family?
14. What are the critical issues in the rehabilitation process which can create the conditions for substance use and abuse?
15. If a person under the influence of drugs or alcohol is injured while riding a motorcycle, who should be responsible for the medical costs? Should insurance be void?
16. Should the manufacturers of beer and spirits be liable for the consequences of use of their products?

References

Abel, E.L. and Ziendenberg, P. (1985) Age, alcohol and violent death: a postmortem study, *J. of Stud. on Alcohol*, 46(3).

Alterman, A.I. and Tarter, R.E. (1985) Relationship between familial alcoholism and brain injury, *J. of Stud. on Alcohol*, 46(3), 256–258.

Anda, R.F., Williamson, D.F., and Remington, P.O. (1988) Alcohol and fatal injuries in the U.S., *J. of the Am. Med. Assoc.*, 33, 132–147.

Beck, R., Marr, K., and Taricone, P. (1991) Identifying and treating clients with physical disabilities who had substance abuse problems, *Rehabil. Educ.*, 5, 131–138.

Benshoff, J.J. and Leal, A. (1990) Substance abuse: challenges for the rehabilitation counseling profession, *J. of Appl. Rehabil. Counseling*, 21(3), 3.

Blackerby, W.F. and Baumgarten, A. (1990) A model treatment program for the head-injured substance abuser: preliminary findings, *J. of Head Trauma Rehabil.*, 5(3), 47–59.

Blair, H.W. (1888) *The Temperance Movement or the Conflict between Man and Alcohol*, William E. Smythe Company, Boston.

Bogner, J. and Lamb-Hart, G. (1995) Did I mention the teeth? *i.e. Magazine*, Ontario Canada Brain Injury Association Journal, Ontario Brain Injury Association, 3(1), 12–15.

Bombardier, C.H., Edhe, D., and Kilmer, J. (1997) Readiness to change alcohol drinking habits after traumatic brain injury, *Arch. of Phys. Med. and Rehabil.*, 78(6), 592–596.

Bombardier, C.H., Kilmer, J., and Edhe, D. (1997) Screening for alcoholism with recent traumatic brain injury, *Rehabil. Psychol.*, 42(4), 259–271.

Bond, M.R. (1986) Neurobehavioral sequelae of closed brain injury, in *Neuropsychological Assessment of Neuropsychiatric Disorders*, Grant, I. and Adams, K., Eds., Oxford University Press, New York.

Bonger, J.A., Corrigan, J.D., Spafford, D.E., and Lamb-Hart, G.L. (1997) Integrating substance abuse treatment and vocational rehabilitation after traumatic brain injury, *J. of Head Trauma*, 12(5), 57–71.

Boros, A., Ed. (1989) Alcohol and the physically impaired, *Alcohol Health and Res. World*, 13(2), 31–36.

Brain Injury Rehabiliation Update (1998) Department of Rehabilitation Medicine, University of Washington, School of Medicine, Seattle, WA, Summer, 9(1).

Bratter, T.E. and Forrest, G.G. (1985) *Alcoholism and Substance Abuse: Strategies for Clinical Intervention*, The Free Press, New York.

Brown, V.B., Ridgely, M.S., Pepper, B., Levine, I.S., and Ryglewicz, H. (1989) The dual crisis: mental illness and substance abuse, present and future directions, *Am. Psychol. Assoc., Inc.*, 44(3), 565–569.

Burke, W.H., Weselowski, M.D., and Guth, W.L. (1988) Comprehensive brain injury rehabilitation: an outcome evaluation, *Brain Injury*, 2, 313–322.

Carey, K.B. (1989). Emerging treatment guidelines for mentally ill chemical abusers, *Hosp. and Community Psychiatr.*, 40, 341–349.

Cherry, L. (1988). Final Report: Bay Area Project on Disabilities and Chemical Dependency, IADD, Hayward, CA.

Corrigan, J.D. (1995) Substance abuse as a mediating factor in outcome from traumatic brain injury, *Arch. of Phys. Med. and Rehabil.*, 76, 302–309.

Corrigan, J.D., Lamb-Hart, G.L., and Rust, E. (1995) A program of interventions for substance abuse following traumatic brain injury, *Brain Injury*, 9(3), 221–236.

Corrigan, J.D., Rust, E., and Lamb-Hart, G.L. (1995) The nature and extent of substance abuse problems among persons with traumatic brain injuries, *J. of Head Trauma Rehabil.*, 10(3), 29–45.

Corrigan, J.D. (1996) The incidence and impact of substance abuse following traumatic brain injury, in *Recovery after Traumatic Brain Injury*, Uzzell, B.P., Stonnington, H.H., and Soronzo, J., Eds., Lawrence Erlbaum Associates, Inc., Hillsdale, NJ.

Corrigan, J.D., Bogner, J.A., and Lamb-Hart, G.L. (1999) Substance abuse and brain injury, in *Rehabiliatation of the Adult and the Child with Traumatic Brain Injury*, 3rd ed., Rosenthal, M., Grifith, E.R., Miller, J.D., and Kreutzer, J., Eds., F.A. Davis, Philadelphia.

Daley, D.C., Moss, H., and Campbell, F. (1987) *Dual Disorders: Counseling Clients with Chemical Dependency and Mental Illness*, Hazelden, Center City, MN.

Dean, J.C., Fos, A.M., and Jensen, W. (1985) Drug and alcohol use by disabled and non-disabled persons: a comparative study, *Int. J. of Addictions*, 20, 629–641.

Delmonico, R., Hanley-Peterson, P., and Englander, J. (1998) Group psychotherapy for persons with traumatic brain injury: management of frustration and substance abuse, *J. of Head Trauma Rehabil.*, 13(6), 10–22.

Dikmen, S., Machmer, J., Donovan, D., Winn, R., and Temkin, N. (1995) Alcohol use before and after traumatic brain injury, *Ann. of Emergency Med.*, 26, 167–176.

Doyle-Pita, D. (1995) *Addictions Counseling*, Crossroads Publishing, New York.

Drake, R.E., Mercer-McFadden, C., Mueser, K.T., McHugo, G.J., and Bond, G.R. (1998) Review of integrated mental health and substance abuse treatment for patients with dual disorders, *Schizophr. Bull.*, 24(4), 589–608.

Fallon, W. (1990) The effect of alcohol in the bloodstream after motor vehicle crash, *Top. in Emergency Med.*, 12(4), 53–56.

Fort, J. (1973) *Alcohol: Our Biggest Drug Problem and Our Biggest Industry*, McGraw-Hill, New York.

Frieden, A. (1990) Substance abuse and disability: the role of the independent living center, *J. of Appl. Rehabil. Counseling*, 21(3), 33–36.

Frisbie, J. H. and Tun, C.G. (1984) Drinking and spinal cord injury, *J. of the Am. Paraplegic Soc.*, 7, 71–73.

Galbraith, S., Murray, W.R., Patel, A.R., and Knill-Jones, R. (1976) The relationship between alcohol and brain injury, and its effects on the conscious level, *Br. J. of Surg.*, 63, 128–130.

Greenbaum, P., Foster-Johnson, L., and Petrilia, A. (1996) Co-occuring addictive and mental disorders among adolescents: prevalence research and further direction, *Am. J. of Orthopsychiatr.*, 66, 1.

Greer, B., Roberts, R., and Jenkins, W. (1990) Substance abuse among clients with other primary disabilities: curricular implications for rehabilitation education, *Rehabil. Educ.*, 4, 33–44.

Greer, B. (1986) Substance abuse among people with disabilities: a problem of too much accessibility, *J. of Rehabil.*, 52, 34–38.

Greer, B. and Walls, R. (1997) Emotional factors involved in substance abuse in a sample of rehabiliation clients, *J. of Rehabil.*, 63(4), 5–8.

Harrison-Felix, C., Zafonte, R., Mann, N., Dijkers, M., Englander, J., and Kreutzer, J. (1998) Brain injury as a result of violence: preliminary findings from the traumatic brain injury model systems, *Arch. of Phys. Med. and Rehabil.*, 79(7), 730–737.

Heinemann, A.W., Keen, M., Donahue, R., and Schnoll, S. (1988) Alcohol use by persons with recent spinal cord injury, *Arch. of Phys. Med. and Rehabil.*, 69, 619–624.

Heinemann, A.W., Doll, M., and Schnoll, S. (1989) Treatment of alcohol abuse in persons with recent spinal cord injury, *Alcohol Health and Res. World*, 13, 110–117.

Heinemann, A.W., Ed. (1993) *Substance Abuse and Disability*, Haworth Press, Binghamton, NY.

Hibbard, M., Uysal, S., Kepler, K., Bogdany, J., and Silver, J. (1998) Axis 1 psychopathology in individuals with traumatic brain injury, *J. of Head Trauma Rehabil.*, 13(4), 24–39.

Hingson, R. and Howland, J. (1987) Alcohol as a risk factor for injury or death resulting from accidental falls: a review of the literature, *J. of Stud. on Alcohol*, 43(3), 212–219.

Huth, J., Maier, R., Simnowitz, D., and Herman, C. (1983) Effect of acute ethanolism on the hospital course and outcome of injured automobile drivers, *The J. of Trauma*, 23, 494–498.

Jaffe, D., Chung, R., and Freidman, L. (1996) Management of portal hypertension and its complications, *Med. Clin. of North Am.*, 80, 121–1034.

Jernigan, D.H. (1991) Alcohol and head trauma: strategies for prevention, *J. of Head Trauma Rehabil.*, 6, 48–60.

Jones, G.A. (1989) Alcohol abuse and traumatic brain damage, *Alcohol Health and Res. World*, 13, 104–109.

Kinney, J. and Leaton, G. (1987) *Loosening the Grip: A Handbook of Alcohol Information*, Times Mirror/Mosby College Publishing, St. Louis.

Kirubakaran, V.R., Kuman, V.N., Powell, B.J., Tyler, A.J., and Armatas, P.J. (1986) Survey of alcohol and drug misuse in spinal cord injured veterans, *J. of Stud. on Alcohol*, 47, 223–227.

Kofoed, L., Kania, J., Walsh, T., and Atkinson, R.M. (1986) Outpatient treatment of patients with substance abuse and coexisting psychiatric disorders, *Am. J. of Psychiatr.*, 143, 867–872.

Kofoed, L. and Keys, A. (1998) Using group therapy to persuade dual-diagnosis patients to seek substance abuse treatment, *Hosp. and Community Psychiatr.*, 39(11), 1209–1214.

Kolakowsky-Hayner, S., Gourley, E., Kreutzer, J., Marwitz, J., Cifu, D., and McKinley, W. (1999) Preinjury substance abuse among persons with brain injury and persons with spinal cord injury, *Brain Injury*, in press.

Krause, J.S. (1992) Delivery of substance abuse services during spinal cord injury rehabilitation, *Neuro Rehabil.*, 2(1), 45–51.

Kreutzer, J.S., Myers, S.L., Harris, J.A., and Zasler, W.D. (1990) Alcohol, brain injury, manslaughter and suicide, *Cognit. Rehabil.*, 8(4), 14–18.

Kreutzer, J.S., Marwitz, J., and Wehman, P.H. (1991) Substance abuse assessment and treatment in vocational rehabilitation for persons with brain injury, *J. of Head Trauma Rehabil.*, 6(3), 12–23.

Kreutzer, J.S., Leininger, B.E., and Harris, J.A. (1989) The evolving role of neuropsychology in community integration, in *Community Integration Following Traumatic Brain Injury*, Kreutzer, J.S. and Wehman, P., Eds., Paul H. Brookes, Baltimore, 49–66.

Kreutzer, J.S. and Harris, J. (1990) Model systems of treatment for alcohol abuse following traumatic brain injury, *Brain Injury*, 4(1), 1–5.

Kreutzer, J.S., Doherty, K.R., Harris, J.A., and Zasler, N.D. (1990) Alcohol use among persons with traumatic brain injury, *J. of Head Trauma Rehabil.*, 5(3), 9–20.

Kreutzer, J.S., Marwitz, J.H., and Witol, A.D. (1995) Interelations between crime, substance abuse, and aggressive behavior among persons with brain injury, *Brain Injury*, 9, 757–768.

Kreutzer, J.S., Witol, A.D., Sander, A.M., Cifu, D.X., Marwitz, J.H., and Delmonico, R.L. (1996) A prospective longitudinal multicenter analysis of alcohol use patterns among persons with traumatic brain injury, *J. of Head Trauma Rehabil.*, 11(5), 58, 59.

Kreutzer, J.S., Witol, A.D., and Marwitz, J.H. (1997) Alcohol and drug use among young persons with traumatic brain injury, in *Childhood Traumatic Brain Injury: Diagnosis, Assessment and Intervention*, Bigler, E., Clark, E., and Farmer, J., Eds., Pro-Ed, Austin, TX, 63–77.

Kreutzer, J. and Sander, A. (1997) Issues in brain injury evaluation and treatment, *Rehabil. Psychol.*, 42(3), 231–239.

Langley, M.J. and Kiley, D.J. (1992) Prevention of substance abuse in persons with neurological disabilities, *Neuro Rehabil.*, 2(1), 52–64.

Langley, M.J. (1991) Preventing post injury alcohol-related problems: a behavioral approach, in *Work Worth Doing: Advances in Brain Injury Rehabil.*, McMahon, B.T. and Shaw, L.R., Eds., Paul M. Deutsch Press, Orlando, FL, 251–275.

Langley, M.J., Lindsay, W.P., Lam, C.S., and Priddy, D.A. (1990) A comprehensive alcohol abuse treatment program for persons with traumatic brain injury, *Brain Injury*, 4(1), 77–86.

Learner, L. (1998) Substance abuse and brain injury, TBI Challenge, Brain Injury Association, Alexandria,VA, 2(6), 5.

Lehman, L., Pilich, A., and Andrews, N. (1994) Neurological disorders resulting from alcoholism, *Alcohol Health and Res. World*, 17, 305–309.

Li, L. and Ford, J. (1998) Illicit drug use by women with disabilities, *The Am. J. on Addictions*, 24(3), 105–118.

Lowenstein, S.R., Weissberg, M., and Terry, D. (1990) Alcohol intoxication, injuries, and dangerous behaviors, and the revolving emergency department door, *J. of Trauma*, 30(10), 1252–1258.

Maio, R., Waller, P., Blow, F., Hill, E., and Singer, K. (1997) Alcohol abuse/dependency in motor vehicle crash victims presenting to the emergency department, *Acad. Emergency Med.*, 4, 4.

McKelvy, M.J., Kane, J.S., and Kellison, K. (1987) Substance abuse and mental illness: double trouble, *J. of Psychosoc. Nursing*, 25(1), 20–25.

Miller, L. (1989) Neuropsychology, personality and substance abuse: implications for brain injury rehabilitation, *Cognit. Rehabil.*, 7(5), 26–31.

Miller, L. (1990) Major syndromes of aggressive behavior following brain injury: an introduction to evaluation and treatment, *Cognit. Rehabil.*, Nov./Dec., 14–19.

Minkoff, K. and Ajilore, C. (1998) Co-occurring psychiatric and substance abuse disorders in managed care systems: standards of care, practice guideline, work-force competencies, and training curricula, Report Center for Mental Health Services Managed Care Initiative, Rockville, MD.

Moore, D. and Seigel, H. (1989) Double trouble: alcohol and other drug use among orthopedically impaired college students, *Alcohol Health and Res. World*, 13(2), 118–123.

Moore, D., Greer, B., and Li, L. (1994) Alcohol and other substance use/abuse among people with disabilities: psychosocial perspective on disability, *J. of Soc. Behavior and Personality*, 9, 369–382.

Moore, D. and Ford, J. (1996) Policy responses to substance abuse and disability: a concept paper, *J. of Disabil. Policy Stud.*, 7(1), 91–106.

Moore, D. and Li, L. (1998) Prevalence and risk factors of illicit drug use by people with disabilities, *The Am. J. on Addictions*, 7(2), 93–102.

Mueser, K. and Fox, L. (1998) Dual diagnosis: how families can help, *J. of the Cal. Alliance for the Mentally Ill*, 9, 53–55.

Murphy, G., Wetzel, R., Robins, E., and McEvoy, L. (1992) Multiple risk factors predict suicide in alcoholism, *Arch. of Gen. Psychiatr.*, 49, 459–463.

National Brain Injury Foundation (1988) National Brain injury Foundation — Professional Council Substance Abuse Task Force White Paper, National Brain injury Foundation, Washington, D.C.

Noble, E.P. (1978) Alcohol and Health, Report No. HE 20.8313:2, U.S. Department of Health, Education, and Welfare, Rockville, MD.

Ohio Valley Center for Brain Injury Prevention and Rehabilitation (1998) Substance Use and Abuse after Brain Injury: A Progammer's Guide, Ohio State University, Columbus, OH.

Peterson, J.B., Rothfleisch, J., Zelazo, P.D., and Pihl, R.O. (1990) Acute alcohol intoxication and cognitive functioning, *J. of Stud. on Alcohol*, 51, 114–122.

Pires, M. (1989) Substance abuse: the silent saboteur in rehabilitation, *Nursing Clinics of N. Am.*, 24(1), 291–296.

Rasmussen, G.A. and DeBoer, R.P. (1981) Alcohol and drug use among clients at a residential vocational rehabilitation center, *Alcohol Health and Res. World*, 5, 48–56.

Rimel, R.W. (1982) Moderate brain injury: completing the clinical spectrum of brain trauma, *Neurosurg.*, 2, 65–73.

Rimel, R.W., Giordani, B.G., Barth, J.T., and Jane, J.A. (1982) Moderate brain injury: completing the clinical spectrum of brain trauma, *Neurosurg.*, 11(3), 344–341.

Rimel, R.W., Giordani, B.G., Barth, J.T., Boll, T.J., and Jane, J.A. (1981) Disability caused by minor brain injury, *Neurosurg.*, 9, 221–228.

Rohe, D.E. and Depompolo, R.W. (1985) Substance abuse policies in rehabilitation medicine departments, *Arch. of Phys. Med. and Rehabil.*, 66, 701–703.

Ruff, R., Marshall, L., Klauber, M., Blunt, B., Grant, I., Foulkes, M., Eisenberg, H., Jane, J., and Marmarou, A. (1990) Alcohol abuse and neurological outcome of the severely head injured, *J. of Head Trauma Rehabil.*, 5(3), 21–31.

Ryan, C. and Butters, N. (1983) Cognitive deficits in alcoholics, in *The Pathogenesis of Alcoholism: Biological Factors*, Kissin, B. and Begleiter, H., Eds., Plenum Press, New York.

Sander, A., Kreutzer, J., and Fernandez, C. (1997) Neurobehavioral functioning, substance abuse and employment after traumatic brain injury: implications for vocational rehabilitation, *J. of Head Trauma Rehabil.*, 12(5), 28–41.

Sander, A., Witol, A., and Kreutzer, J. (1997) Alcohol use after traumatic brain injury: concordance of patients' and relatives' reports, *Arch. of Phys. Med. and Rehabil.*, 78(2), 138–142

SARDI (1996) Substance Abuse, Disability and Vocational Rehabilitation, Research and Training Center on Drugs and Disability, Wright State School of Medicine, Dayton, OH, 2.

Schuckit, M.A. (1986) Primary men alcoholics with histories of suicide attempts, *J. of Stud. on Alcoholism*, 47, 78–81.

Schuckit, M.A. (1995a) Alcohol related disorders, in Comprehensive Textbook of Psychiatry, 6th ed., Kaplan, H.I. and Sadock, B.J., Eds., Williams & Wilkins, Baltimore.

Schuckit, M.A. (1995b) *Drug and Alcohol Abuse: A Clinical Guide to Diagnosis and Treatment*, 4th ed., Plenum Press, New York.

Schuckit, M.A. (1996) Alcohol, anxiety and depressive disorders, *Alcohol Health and Res. World*, 20, 81–86.

Sciacca, K. and Thompson, C. (1996) Program development and integrated treatment across systems for dual diagnosis: mental illness, drug addiction, and alcoholism, *The J. of Ment. Health Adm.*, 23(3), 288–297.

Seaton, J.D. and David, C.O. (1990) Family role in the substance abuse and traumatic brain injury rehabilitation, *J. of Head Trauma Rehabil.*, 5(3), 41–46.

Shapiro, R. (1982) Clinical approaches to family violence, *The Fam. Ther. Coll.*, Aspen, Rockville.

Shipley, R., Taylor, S., and Falvo, D. (1990) Concurrent evaluation and rehabilitation of alcohol abuse and trauma, *J. of Appl. Rehabil. Counseling*, 21(3), 37–39.

Soderstrom, C.A. and Cowley, R.A. (1987) A national alcohol and trauma center survey, *Arch. of Surg.*, 122, 1071–1087.

Solomon, D. and Sparadeo, F.R. (1992) Effects of substance use on persons with traumatic brain injury, *Neuro Rehabil.*, 2(1), 16–26.

Sparadeo, F.R. and Gill, D. (1989) Effects of prior alcohol use on brain injury recovery, *J. of Head Trauma Rehabil.*, 4(1), 75–82.

Sparadeo, F.R., Strauss, D., and Barth, J.T. (1990) The incidence, impact and treatment of substance abuse on head trauma rehabilitation, *J. of Head Trauma Rehabil.*, 5(3), 1–8.

Sparadeo, F.R. Strauss, D., and Kapsales, K.B. (1992) Substance abuse, brain injury, and family adjustment, *Neuro Rehabil.*, 2(1), 65–73.

Sparadeo, F.R., Barth, J.T., Stout, C.E., Levitt, J.L., and Ruben, D.H. (1992) Addiction and traumatic brain injury, in *Handbook for Assessing and Treating Addictive Disorders*, Stout, C.E., Levitt, J.L., and Ruben, D.H., Eds., Greenwood Press, New York.

Sternberg, D.W. (1986) Dual diagnosis: addiction and affective disorders, *The Psychiatr. Hosp.*, 20, 71–77.

Straussman, J. (1985) Dealing with double disabilities: alcohol use in the club, *Psychosoc. Rehabil. J.*, 8(3), 8–14.

Tate, D. (1993) Alcohol use among spinal cord injured patients, *Am. J. of Phys. Med. and Rehabil.*, 72(4), 192–195.

Teplin, L.A., Abram, K.M., and Stuart, K. (1989) Blood alcohol level among emergency room patients: a multivariate analysis, *J. of Stud. on Alcohol*, 50(3), 441–447.

Tobis, J.S., Puri, K.B., and Sheridan, J. (1982) Rehabilitation of the severely brain injured patient, *Scand. J. of Rehabil. Med.*, 14, 655–667.

Waller, J.A. (1990) Management issues for trauma patients with alcohol, *J. of Trauma*, 30(12), 1548–1553.

Waller, P., Blow, F., Maio, R., Singer, K., Hill, E., and Schaffer, N. (1997) Crash characteristics and injuries of victims impaired by alcohol versus illicit drugs, *Accident Anal. and Prev.*, 29(6), 817–827.

Weiss, R. and Frankel, R. (1989) Closed brain injury and substance abuse: the dual misdiagnosis, *Prof. Counselor*, 3(4), 49–51.

Wolkstein, E. and Moore, D. (1996) Substance Abuse, Disability and Vocational Rehabilitation, Training Manual, SARDI, Wright State School of Medicine, Dayton, OH.

Woosley, E.E. (1981) Psycho-social aspects of substance abuse among the physically disabled, *Alcohol Health and Res. World*, U.S. Department of Health and Human Services, Washington, D.C.

Yates, W.R., Meller, W., and Toughton, E.P. (1987) Behavioral complications of alcoholism, *Am. Fam. Phys.*, 35(3), 171–175.

Zasler, N.D. (1991) Update on pharmacology: neuromedical aspects of alcohol use following traumatic brain injury, *J. of Head Trauma Rehabil.*, 6(4), 78–80.

Zink, B., Maio, R., and Chen, B. (1996) Alcohol, central nervous system injury, and time to death in fatal motor vehicle crashes, *Alcoholism: Clin. and Exp. Res.*, 20(9).

chapter eleven

Caregiving and respite care

Perspective

Caregiving and respite care are vital forces in coping with the complex demands of an illness–disability experience, especially when considering those living with brain injuries. The challenge is attending to the complex needs of the patient while shoring up the resources and meeting the current and future needs of the family. This is not an easy task and it presents many problems.

Some of the major problems encountered by caregivers are identified by Kahana et al. (1994):

1. Coping with increased needs of the dependent family member caused by physical and/or mental illnesess
2. Coping with disruptive behaviors especially those associated with cognitive disorders or mental illness such as dementia or schizophrenia
3. Restrictions on social or leisure activities
4. Infringement of privacy
5. Disruption of household and work routines
6. Conflicting multiple role demands
7. Lack of support and assistance from other family members
8. Disruptions of family roles and relationships
9. Lack of sufficient assistance from human service agencies and agency professionals

Traditionally caregiving has been viewed as an expectation from those who are in traditonal caregiving roles, e.g., parents, spouses, significant others, children, relatives, etc. More recently caregiving has been extended to those persons who provide such care on a compensated or volunteer basis. Such caregiving has become the focus of ongoing discussion and debate (Angell, 1999; Arno, Levine, and Memmott, 1999; Levine, 1998, 1999; Levine and Zuckerman, 1999).

This urgent situation is captured and presented by Levine (1999):

> Family caregivers must be supported, because the
> health care system cannot exist without them. Exhaust-
> ed caregivers may become care recipients, leading to a
> further, often preventable, drain on resources" (p. 1559).

For some families caregiving can be a source of joy. For others caregiving can be a stressful process. For most families the reality is somewhere in between. Biegel (1995) states:

> The provision of care to a family member who has a
> chronic illness implies a significant expenditure of time
> and energy over potential long periods of time, in-
> volves tasks that may be unpleasant and uncomfort-
> able, is likely to be nonsymmetrical (the caregiver often
> gives more than he or she receives in return from the
> care recipient) and is often a role that has not been
> anticipated.

He further states that, "Research on the effects of caregiving shows very clearly that caregiving is not without costs to the caregiver. Many families report caregiving to be an emotional, physical and at times, financial burden" (p. 146).

Even successful caregiving can be like a double-edged sword. Some caregivers are able to negotiate the demands of caregiving because they see it as time limited, with an end in sight. For others the process is complicated by their need to hold on and make things better, all the while feeling dis-tressed because they want to let go and get on with their lives.

In discussing brain injury and caregiving, several concepts should be considered:

- No person or family is ever prepared for the reality of a brain injury experience.
- Brain injury changes a family and challenges its resources.
- A brain injury brings out the best and worst in people.
- Brain injury can deplete family resources and create them.
- By intent or default, often the only support available is the family.
- Not everyone has a family to rely on.
- Not all families are capable of responding to the caregiving needs of a brain-injured family member.
- New skills are needed by the family to meet the ongoing challenges created by brain injury.
- Not everyone is going to improve.
- Sometimes the best programs do not make a difference.

- Coping with brain injury is an ongoing developmental process for the patient and family.
- Respite care often makes the difference between coping and deteriorating.
- Not all family members love or hate the person with brain injury.
- Often families survive by creating hope based upon desperation and not reality.
- Existing health care resources can help and hinder adjustment.
- Financial resources can solve or create problems.

These points are made as selected examples of issues that can be considered and handled if the family is going to achieve survival, development, enrichment, and a reasonable quality of life. Kosciulek and Lustig (1998) have discussed family adaptation to brain injury in the context of family stress. Lustig (1999) discussed the role of stress and its impact on the family:

> Family stress is the result of an imbalance between the demands placed on the family and capabilities of the family to deal with the stressor. When the demand-capability imbalance is pronounced, the family may experience maladjustment. The ability of the family to successfully adjust to a stressor is determined by the family's vulnerability, resources, appraisal, problem solving and coping (p. 26).

However, in this time of managed care and managed cost, policy makers and systems are expecting that families should be in a position to assume more involved roles with little or no compensation or acknowledgement. This is presumptuous and potentially risky for all involved.

Presenting both the objective facts and subjective realities, Levine (1999) states:

> Health care policy makers and analysts rarely consider the impact of these (financial) incentives on the 25 million unpaid, informal caregivers in the United States, who get little from the system in return for the estimated $196 billion a year in labor they provide" (p. 1587).

She further states:

> I feel abandoned by a health care system that commits resources and rewards to rescuing the injured and ill but then consigns such patients and their families to the black hole of chronic custodial care (p. 1588).

An important question to address is: how can the family be supported and have access to those resources that acknowledge the value of their contributions? If families are not able to do this, someone will have to back-fill the void — often at inflated and unreasonable costs. At times reason does not prevail. It seems that there is more of a willingness to spend money and allocate resources for disaster relief rather than disaster privation. The result is "the hole is too deep and the ladder is too short." This is especially true for those families responsible for the caregiving of a brain-injured member during the home re-entry process.

While recognizing the increased opportunities that have resulted from deinstitutionalization, Mesibov and Price (1995) remind us that new problems and challenges for the community and family have been created. Families need their injured family member to have 24-hour care, and respite care is critical in helping families cope with the stress related to the caregiving process. The complexities of the problems have become a focal point for policy makers (Angell, 1999; Arno et al., 1999; Kane and Penrod, 1995) and caregivers who are often lost in the process (Levine, 1998, 1999; Houts et al., 1996).

The reality is that family members may be able to tolerate a life of self-denial for a few days or weeks, but they won't be able to endure a regimen of emotional and social deprivation indefinitely without becoming physically ill or emotionally wrought (Oddy et al., 1978).

Addressing the changes consequent to caregiving at home, Deboskey (1996) states, "There is no question that bringing your loved one home changes your life and impacts upon your mental health status" (p. 45).

While it is conceptually easy to understand the philosophies and principles of caregiving, it's more difficult to implement. This is often due to the complex emotional forces that can influence the process and the historical reality that impacts the ability of families to assume the caregiving role.

For example, a spouse who believes he has a quality relationship with his spouse may be better able to make the transition from marital partner to caregiver than a spouse who is in a toxic relationship with his spouse and who is looking for a way out and not a long-term commitment to a stressful caregiving role.

Knop et al. (1998) discusses the relationship between coping and the quality of marital relationships as they influence the caregiving process of spouses with Alzheimer's Disease. The quality of the marital relationship has a role in determining how the caregiver will respond to the demands of the caregiving process (Morris et al., 1988). In long-term care situations the caregiving burden can become more difficult because unresolved issues and marital discord intensify as the needs of the recipient of care increase (Wright, 1993).

Having a strong marriage or relationship is not a guarantee that the transition to caregiving will be successful. However, a solid relationship means that there is a greater probability that caregiving can be sustained. Under difficult circumstances, it is important to note that many solid relationships can be fractured while some marginal or problematic relationships can be refocused and enhanced by an illness, disability, or brain injury experience.

This is an important point when planning for intervention and support because a caregiver may appear to be coping well at one point and be at great risk at another. Understanding how families cope and survive have been the focus of McCubbin et al. (1996) regarding the resiliency model of family stress.

Chwalisz (1992, 1996) explored the concepts of subjective burden and perceived stress as they relate to spouses of persons with brain injuries. The importance of family burden in the caregiving process is stressed by Allen et al. (1994).

Gillen et al. (1998) emphasize that in addition to adverse outcomes such as suicide, hospitalization, and divorce, depression may be associated with impaired caregiving, or caregiving that is so overwhelming it is not in the best interest of the patient. This is an important point when there is the expectation that families will devote their resources and engage in the demands of caregiving when they have not been given the support they need to give care. A key point made by Gillen et al. (1998) is that even if supports are in place during hospitalization or rehabilitation, they may not be the best fit for the caregiver. They say, "The most intensive support services, typically provided to caretakers during the inpatient phase of reha-bilitation, may simply not match well with the course over which depression develops" (p. 41).

Need

In order to better understand the family's need for support for caregiving and respite care, it is important to recognize the developmental process associated with a brain injury. Since brain injuries do not impact everyone at the same point in the life spans, it is imperative that caregiving and respite care programs have the potential to respond to an evolving need system. While the nature of the brain injury plays a major role in the determination of need, consideration must also be given to the complexities of the emerging interaction between the family and the patient.

First, the needs of the family member living with the brain injury vary according to the intensity of the physical and emotional aspects of the dis-ability, age of the person, the role in the family, and the potential to maintain a degree of self dignity based on what was, what is, and what will be. Second, the needs of the family vary according to structure, resources, traditions, developmental stage, and ability to access support and accept the demands of the brain injury experience.

These individual and familial needs, however, do not exist in isolation from the community, society, or health care system. As DeJong et al. (1990) state:

> If the responsibility for persons with brain injury were
> truly a shared obligation, the perceived burden of ev-
> eryday caring by families would lighten substantially
> while the increased burden on the community and
> society would remain manageable (p. 21).

While family history, personal experiences, and role models can be important factors in creating the perspective needed to meet the demands of a brain
injury experience, the outcomes are not always ideal. For example, if the
caring for a head-injured family member has created a significant amount of
family stress, the family may decide that they will never place themselves in
a similar situation. However, some families may be able to recognize why
the situation is so stressful and make changes which can reduce stress and
make the future situations more bearable, functional, and positive.

Frequently, the major stressor in the brain injury experience is the dramatic change of roles. These role shifts can occur when an affectionate,
responsible spouse becomes a demanding, irresponsible patient and the
loving, caring spouse becomes a resentful caregiver who sees caregiving
more as a curse than an opportunity. Rosenthal (1987) addresses the intensity
of the situation when he states:

> Spouses may feel as though they are living with
> strangers; relatives may reject the injured member be-
> cause they do not recognize and/or understand how
> to deal with subtle neurobehavioral disturbances.
> Friends may vanish due to the head injured patient's
> personality change, physical or mental limitation, im-
> paired social skills, or inability to "fit in" with the
> group (p. 55).

The following examples may provide a perspective on the stressors
related to caregiving which could warrant respite care:

1. A husband with a brain injury who cannot regulate bodily functions
   and has to be constantly supervised. Enormous stress is placed upon
   the wife and children because he acts like a six-year-old child who
   has a severe disability and requires ongoing care.
2. The elderly parent who has a child with a severe developmental
   disability and was able to manage with the help of her son until he
   sustained a brain injury and became a patient rather than a caregiver.
3. A woman who has multiple sclerosis and cannot get help from her
   husband who was brain injured. This is complicated by the constant
   turnover of workers and lack of a supportive family.

What these examples have in common is the intensity of a situation
which has resulted in increased family stress, creating the potential for accel-

erated familial deterioration. Respite care in such situations enables the family to create a pause in the caregiving process and develop a different frame of reference. As a result, family members are able to renegotiate their familial roles and establish new ones which are more conducive to coping, rejuvenation, and survival.

Families may be put in a position of having to choose between their emotional and physical stability and the care of a member having a brain injury. For example, some family members may want to keep the person at home while others may want to place the person in a long-term care facility. In such cases, respite care options can often make the difference between a family's ability to make lifetime care choices from a position of strength rather than default. The complexity of these choices is addressed by Jarman and Stone (1989) when they state:

> Some parents may find they simply cannot provide the care their loved one needs, no matter how hard they try. At this point they agonize over the right decision, and are forced to acknowledge that they cannot make it "all better" for their injured child. Considering placement and alternative living options becomes a very difficult decision-making process for these parents (p. 32).

While never easy, the caregiving process can be supported by the existence of respite care options. In effect, caregiving and respite care are synergistic processes that can make the difference for those families in desperate need of support, replenishment, and validation.

Respite care

Respite care is emerging as a vital force which is often the only buffer between the family and the ravages of illness and disability (Botuck and Winsberg, 1991; Grant and Mcgrath, 1990; Lawton et al., 1989; Marks, 1987; Pearson and Deitrick, 1989; Rimmerman, 1989).

A major problem with brain injury treatment and rehabilitation is that many of the difficulties encountered by persons experiencing brain injuries and their families are not directly caused by the brain injuries, but by the lack of respite care and other services (Brown and McCormick, 1988; Campbell, 1988; Graff and Minnes, 1989; Ridley, 1989). This situation exists because health care and rehabilitation systems are designed to provide treatment based on the assumption that at some point the person, family, or significant other will develop the physical, financial, and emotional resources necessary to deal with the torrent of demands following a brain injury. The reality is that many people do not have families or significant others who have unlimited emotional, financial, and physical resources to respond to the evolving challenges of a brain injury experience. As DeJong et al. (1990) state:

Furthermore, some head-injured persons have a supportive family, and some have no family; some are
employable, and some are not; some have access to
financial resources, and some have no resources.
Therefore, the extent to which individuals must rely
on family and society for support depends largely on
their personal conditions and socioeconomic circumstances (p. 12).

It is imperative that the respite care needs of individuals and families
be taken into consideration. Hegeman (1987) states:

The traumatically brain-injured client is not the only
victim; the family and/or significant others suffer as
well. Disruption in the lifestyle and the emotional
strain on the family caused by the trauma result in
complex, long-standing problems.

A similar point is made by Armstrong (1991) who states:

Without the day to day experience of the patient's
irresponsibility, impulsivity, or other problems, or of
the duties, other relatives can easily misperceive the
caretaker as being too protective or restrictive, or too
neglectful or uncaring. Examples of this are unending,
and even those professionals who are most committed
or most caring can make these mistakes. Only those
who have experienced the daily vigilances of care and
worry are likely to be fully grateful and emotionally
supportive of the family's accomplishments in foster-
ing the patient's improvements (p. 20).

Considering the mission of caregiving and respite care, it is important
to evaluate how it is defined. Just as there is variability in the populations
served, there are differences in the definitions of respite care. In their out-
standing book, Cohen and Warren (1985) provide the following statement:

The definition of respite care as "the temporary care of
a disabled individual for the purpose of providing relief to the primary caregiver" seems straightforward
and noncontroversial. However, in practice, there is
considerable variation in the interpretation of the scope
of services to be called respite care. One of these vari-
ations concerns the distinction between intermittent
and ongoing services. Virtually all definitions of respite
care include the idea of temporary services (p. 26).

The problem with a time-limited definition of respite care is that the needs, problems, and concerns of both the patient and family may fluctuate and exist over a lifetime. This is especially true for the family of the person challenged by a brain injury who has long-term needs and short-term resources.

Respite care is defined by Pullo and Hahn (1979) as:

> The temporary and periodic provision of a range of services which prevent individual and family break-down by relieving the caretaker of stress by giving continuous support and/or care to a dependent indi-vidual. These services are not meant to replace other specialized services provided to an individual in need of care (p. 1).

What is significant about this definition is that it conveys a sensitivity to the consequences of unchecked demands made on the family and recog-nizes that a family can be overwhelmed if consistent help is not provided. While the definitions of respite care focus upon the importance of providing relief for the family or caregiver, they also address the importance of avail-able respite care programs.

Theoretically, the availability of such programs should reflect a match between need and resources. Unfortunately, the need most often is in excess of the resources. This may create stress and frustration on the part of those caregivers who are in desperate need of such services. The need for pro-grams is stated by Waaland and Kreutzer (1988) who say that traditional respite care programs "are frequently unavailable to the child with a trau-matic brain injury."

Even if the basic roles and functions of these systems are distinct from those of the family, these systems should be complementary to the respite care goals and familial needs and not adversarial to them. Unfortunately, most health care and political systems are burdened by policies and finances while consumers of respite care are often more concerned with emotional survival and quality of life. This point is made by Durgin (1989) when he states:

> It is critical that family members be aware of their limitations and not feel pressured to take on too much responsibility. Typically, there are a large number of professionals involved in rehabilitation because it is too extreme a challenge for one to "shoulder it all." Families should be sure to say "no" when they cannot take on more and should also let it be known when they would like to be more involved (p. 22).

For families with a character-altered brain-injured member, the issue of respite care is cast in the shadow of an often harsh reality. In this situation, there is an intensification of the responsibilities and consequences of care. Rosenthal and Young (1988) state:

> The chronic nature of the brain injury will prohibit the family from returning to the kind of stability that was characteristic of its functioning prior to the injury. As the family cares for the characterologically altered family member, each person's own emotional and developmental needs become secondary to the management of the brain-injured person within the family (p. 45).

Gender issues and role flexibility

The need for respite care does not differentiate between the gender of the patient and the primary caregiver. Traditionally, the woman has been designated by choice, tradition, or default, to be the provider of "nurturance and care" (Zeigler, 1989). In effect, women often become the caregivers even if they are not the best people for the job. Their efforts and energies may be better placed in other areas.

While there have been gains made in the emergence of new roles for both women and men, there is still concern regarding making the role modifications necessary to respond to the specific needs of a loved one or the complex demands of the respite care process (Stroker, 1983). Therefore, role flexibility is key to ability to alter personal goals, aspirations, and needs for the benefit of the total family system. While difficult in the best of circumstances, role flexibility is almost impossible when elements of personal and familial dysfunction foster role rigidity, interpersonal stress, and pervasive chaos. Consequently, there are few families that can make the transitions from wellness to state of loss and respond constructively if their prior interactions have been dysfunctional. Families who work together, who care about each other, and who have functional role models often make the adjustments which are helpful. As Waaland and Kreutzer (1988) state: "It is thus important that clinicians help families to mobilize effective resources and avoid mutual blaming or unhealthy family realignments that preclude marital health or clear generational boundaries" (p. 57).

Brain injury and respite care

The need for support and respite care is due to the fact that families living brain injury experiences are challenged by long-term situations which may last lifetimes. Acute illness has a built-in respite due to a time limitation while chronic conditions have expanding and long-term demands which can intensify the need for respite care.

There is an added stressor for families when the family member's behavior becomes destructive, aggressive, and dangerous. The person changed by brain injury is perceived as a stranger whose behavior makes an out-of-home placement attractive and home care problematic. Families are so burdened and frustrated that they have "burnout," and make alternate living arrangements based on their frustration and desperation. Often families are reluctant to seek help until they are at the point of physical, financial, and emotional exhaustion, as Waaland and Kreutzer (1988) state: "Prolonged use of maladaptive coping strategies and persistent feelings of helplessness are related to patient confusion, marital conflict, and parental overprotection or inconsistencies" (p. 57).

At this point, great damage has been done and a comprehensive intervention program must be instituted to try to stabilize the patient and the family. This can be achieved through a combination of direct services and seminars which provide skills and peer support.

Not only does respite care help families cope with the challenges of brain injury, it helps the injured persons. Their basic needs are met by the respite care process and they are afforded the chance for "non-maintenance interaction" with their families.

While priority is placed on keeping the person in the community with his or her family, not all communities can provide significant support; some families do not want to while others feel that they cannot take care of the family member.

Though respite care should be a component of a comprehensive intervention, treatment, and rehabilitation model, attention must be given to the multi-dimensional problems that families often face, such as role fatigue, stress, the need for rejuvenation, and the importance of maintaining quality of life. DeJong, Batavia, and Williams (1990) address this point when they state:

> Provision of respite care cannot be addressed by the family, which needs temporary relief from the situation, nor by society, which typically is too removed from the situation to provide humane care. Respite care, and other services such as grocery shopping and housekeeping, may be provided effectively by members of the community (p. 17).

Conclusion

Effective, relevant, and accessible systems of caregiving and respite care help families replace desperation with hope, nothingness with dreams, and isolation with support.

While it would be wonderful if no child, adult, or family had to deal with the ravages of brain injury, life, unfortunately, does not always conform to such aspirations. When brain injury occurs it is often an unending familial nightmare that depletes resources, insults dignity, and often pushes the family to the brink of desperation. Sometimes they survive. At other times, however, the outcome is more disappointing.

The enormity of brain injury is so pervasive that coping with it cannot be the sole responsibility of the family. Therefore, it is imperative that health care professionals be aware of the complexities surrounding the brain injury experience and how it impacts the family. As Rosenthal and Young (1988) state, "Failure to understand the family dynamics following brain injury and to provide the appropriate intervention is likely to limit the potential success of any rehabilitation program" (p. 42).

When discussing the differential impact of brain injury, we must be aware that the resources, problems, needs, and dreams are as different as snowflakes. While the element of individuality is the key to emotional survival, it must be fueled by the commonality which all challenged people and their families share. This commonality is the active ingredient which can enable people to negotiate the challenges of brain injuries by recognizing they are not alone and that respite care services are available to them. It is unfortunate when pain and frustration are increased by the ignorance of resources and models. One explanation for this lack of awareness is that in the midst of a trauma, people are so devastated that they are unable to identify the systems designed to help them.

The value of respite care and self-help organizations is that they enable families to maximize their chances for survival when challenged by brain injuries. Why should people in extreme need feel isolated? Can we not learn from each other, share mutual strengths, and create an environment that facilitates a reasonable quality of life?

Respite care programs are meeting the important needs of families coping with illnesses or disabilities. They represent proven ways to decrease pressures on families challenged by the demands of caregiving (Mesibov and Price, 1995).

Brain injury has the power to limit those affected by it and fragment the family. Effective caregiving and accessible respite care have the potential to put illness, disability, and brain injury into perspective and create options so that families can live as fully as possible. Brain injury is not a trauma that negates humanity, but rather it is a life experience that gives people a chance to demonstrate how caring, committed, and realistic they are.

The following personal statement, *Things Change, A Friend's Perspective* explores the complexity and evolution of a friendship over many years.

Personal statement

Things change, a friend's perspective

Michelle was born before her mother completed her college degree, and two sons followed soon after. Both boys had behavioral problems at school, partially due to learning disabilities and possible attention deficit disorders. The family valued education and both parents were very involved in their children's academic development. They pushed the school system to provide specialized teaching services for their boys. The parents recognized that their boys were bright and hoped they'd be successful in school. Their daughter was doing very well in school. The parents were also involved in all other aspects of their children's lives.

Michelle's parents were distant from their own families and beginning with their sons' difficulties in school, they adopted an us-against-them attitude toward people outside the family. The boys continued to get into trouble in school and with the police for minor antics. The parents were always willing to defend their sons and neither son hesitated to turn to his parents for help. Their daughter continued to do well in school and she stayed out of trouble with the police, although she had adopted a fearless attitude toward authority figures after witnessing her parents defend her brothers many times.

Months after graduating from school, Michelle was severely injured while she was a passenger on a motorcycle. Initially there was little hope for her survival. She had extensive internal injuries and a severe brain injury. When it became more certain that she would live, there was very little hope that she would be able to function effectively. During the acute phase of the injury, the parents kept an around-the-clock vigil at Michelle's bedside. Her mother left her job in order to stay at the hospital full time. At no time did either parent ask family or friends for help, and they rejected help from friends when it was offered. In the eyes of many, they were hyper-functional and very capable to manage all their affairs. The boys suffered greatly by the impact of their sister's injuries and the absence of their parents and began to get into more trouble with the local police. The older son had been using drugs for many years and his drug use increased.

Michelle remained in the acute phase of her injuries for almost a year. She suffered many complications. During this year, friends of her parents never saw nor heard from them and all offers of help were politely rejected. It was determined that Michelle would go to a rehabilitation hospital while she was still on a ventilator. Because of the extent of her head and spinal cord injuries, it was certain that she would never walk. She would have very limited control over her arms. She might learn to speak again, but only after intensive speech therapy. While Michelle was in the rehabilitation hospital her parents visited every day, but they no longer remained at her bedside around-the-clock. Their anxiety had been soothed by a speech therapist who had taken the time to answer their questions and address their concerns. Michelle's mother was able to return to work part-time and spend some time with her youngest son. The family continued to reject help from friends, but began to attend some social functions. Michelle remained in the rehabilitation hospital for 18 months during which time her parents prepared their home for her return. Michelle was quadriplegic with a spastic paralysis, had severe cognitive difficulties, and spoke incomprehensively. Michelle's brother was very much against Michelle's homecoming. He feared the loss of his parents again and was furious with Michelle because of her disabilities. Again, Michelle's mother left work to be with her daughter. She learned all the nursing skills needed to care for Michelle, and her husband helped with all the heavy tasks like lifting and bathing.

Michelle had been home for over 3 years when her mother suffered a nearly fatal heart attack. For many years, her mother had been cautioned to take care of herself and her heart condition. The heart attack forced her to give up some of the care she had been providing. Following the heart attack, Michelle hired a personal care attendants (P.C.A.) to provide for her physical needs. During the two years that Michelle had been home, her speech and cognitive abilities improved while her physical disabilities remained the same. Although her family had often rejected outside help, Michelle welcomed it. She had always been a very social person and she struggled to rebuild a social life. This rebuilding began with the hiring of P.C.A. The first hired was a woman she had been friendly with in high school. Together, with the P.C.A., Michelle began to get out of the house more often. She began to struggle for independence from her mother who wanted to spend all her time with Michelle, although she was unable to provide much of the physical care. Michelle wanted to be able to build a life for herself which included partying with friends her own age. It was now 6 years since the accident and few of Michelle's friends came around. Michelle struggled to gain acceptance but was unable to run with the crowd she had socialized with before the accident. Michelle's speech was still very difficult to understand and she continued to have cognitive difficulties which caused her friends great discomfort.

Nine years after the accident, her mother died of a massive stroke at age 53. The boys, both of whom had been outside the family for years, returned for the funeral. After years of isolation, the funeral brought family and friends back together. Both sons moved back into town shortly after their mother's death. Michelle continued to have most of her needs met by paid professional staff instead of family members. Two years later, her father remarried and his new wife was willing to help the family with Michelle's needs.

Today, Michelle complains of feeling lonely because of the absence of past friends. Her older brother spends more time with her these days. She manages some of her feelings of grief and anger by using drugs and alcohol which her brother supplies. She says getting high helps her when she feels low. She doesn't see her drug use as a problem. Television is a constant companion; she is addicted to soap operas. Michelle never watched television before her injury; she believed most of the shows were written for idiots. She used to love to read but no longer knows how. Recently she discovered books on tape and she enjoys these a great deal. Michelle is able to ask for help and attempts to stay connected with people outside her family.

Thinking back, I must admit that there were years when I didn't visit Michelle at all. The times I did visit were very difficult for me. First of all, the visits always took place in her parents' home. Before the accident, we never spent any time together in our parents' homes. I felt even more uncomfortable because I believed that her parents were angry with me for not visiting more and because I reminded them of Michelle before the accident.

I never knew what to talk about when I was there. I didn't want to talk about my life and all the things I was doing because Michelle could do none of these things. Michelle's personality seemed changed. She was no longer mischievous. Earlier in our friendship, I admired her ability to create fun in almost every situation and her sense of adventure.

One afternoon, about 7 years after the accident, I was visiting with Michelle while her mother was out of the house. As soon as her mother left the house, Michelle asked me if I wanted to smoke some pot. We did and drank a few beers. We had a lot of fun that afternoon. Afterwards, I worried about whether or not it was okay that we partied together. Before the accident, Michelle and I drank every time we were together and now, while I wanted her to feel good and have fun, I worried about the effects of drinking and drugs on her health. Shortly after that, I entered treatment for my own addiction problems and didn't see Michelle for a couple of years. Now when we get together, usually over holidays, we talk about our growing families, our nieces and nephews. Being an aunt is one thing that we have in common and it's a source of joy for both of us.

The years of isolation might have been avoided if the family had been able to trust the assistance of helping professionals. Because of their difficulty with trust even before the accident, it would have taken extraordinary sensitivity on the part of the team working with the family. After years of isolation and chaos, the family is able to function reasonably well today. The boys both have families, and they are very involved with their sister and father. Michelle loves being an aunt; she spends most of her money on clothes and toys for her nephews and niece. She is learning to read again and spends a lot of time reading children's books to them. She has a role in the family again which gives her life purpose and meaning.

Today my relationship with Michelle is more comfortable than it had been in the 15 years since the accident. She continues to get better slowly and we can spend quality time together, boasting about our nieces and nephews. For years I had difficulty knowing what to talk about because I feared anything I'd say about my life would remind her of her loss. Her family was somewhat hostile toward me for years because I didn't visit often enough. I reminded the parents of what they had hoped for Michelle. They are no longer angry, and it is much easier to visit the family home. They are working their way through their losses and they are able to manage the grief that they continue to experience. In almost every way, the family is a functional unit who cares for each other and helps each other weather the difficulties of life and the losses of their dreams. I guess things change.

Discussion questions on the personal statement

1. How does managing and advocating for children who have behavioral problems prepare or not prepare parents to cope with a child with a brain injury?

2. How does the fact that Michelle was injured on a motorcycle influence the coping of the parents?
3. Is having a daughter who survived an accident with little hope for recovery a burden or challenge to this family?
4. What is your reaction to the statement, "The parents kept an around-the-clock vigil at Michelle's bedside?"
5. How can help be offered when families do not want it?
6. How can siblings who "suffer greatly" be supported during the treatment and rehabilitation process?
7. What are the issues and complications generated by Michelle's brain and spinal cord injuries?
8. What response would be helpful to Michelle's brother, who did not want to be displaced by her?
9. What are the issues generated by Michelle's mother's near fatal heart attack?
10. Why did the death of Michelle's mother bring the family together?
11. Is Michelle's use of drugs a problem?
12. If your best friend was in a situation similar to Michelle's, how long would you want to or be able to maintain a relationship — 5, 10, 15 years?

Set 15. How can I help?

Perspective

A characteristic of most suffering is that it is done alone. This is especially true when families are forced to retreat from society and focus all of their energies on the caregiving process. A major tenet of respite care is that the more a burden is shared, the more bearable it becomes.

Exploration

1. Do you know a family dealing with a brain injury? Have you considered reaching out and providing support?
2. Would you respond differently if the patient was a child?
3. If you belong to a religious organization, can you identify how this organization demonstrates the principles of becoming involved, and taking care of people in this life and the next?

Set 16. Who needs this kind of help?

Perspective

When families are in a state of crisis, they need to be listened to, responded to, and treated with sensitivity, caring, and respect. Often the stress of health care and rehabilitation environments creates a situation in which professional and non-professional staff do not provide help but rather create pain with insensitive remarks.

Exploration

List from your personal and/or professional frame of reference examples of how health care and human service professionals have and have not been helpful in dealing with the impacts of brain injuries. For example, a helpful response might be: it is not easy, but we will be there to help. A response that might not be helpful is: after all, your daughter was an alcoholic who should not have been driving.

Additional discussion questions

1. Who should provide respite care in your community?
2. Should respite care be paid for by insurance?
3. Should families be financially compensated for the home care of family members with brain injuries?
4. What would you consider adequate respite care for a family who has a five-year-old child with a brain injury and a parent with terminal cancer?
5. List the important components of a respite care program designed to meet the needs of families challenged by brain injuries.
6. Should individuals or families be legally forced to provide respite care for family members?
7. What would be your reaction to a proposal which suggested that all religious facilities should provide respite care services for the community?
8. How would you challenge the position that states respite care is a luxury, which should not be considered an integral part of the discharge plan?
9. What are the criteria you would use to decide if a family needed respite care?

References

Allen, K., Linn, R., Gutierrez, H., and Willer, B. (1994) Family burden following traumatic brain injury, *Rehabil. Psychol.*, 39(1), 29–48.

Angell, M. (1999) The American health care system revisited — a new series, *New England J. of Med.*, 340, 48.

Armstrong, C. (1991) Emotional changes following brain injury: psychological and neurological components of depression, denial and anxiety, *J. of Rehabil.*, June, 14–17.

Arno, P., Levine, C., and Memmott, M. (1999) The economic value of informal caregiving, *Health Aff.*, 18(2), 182–188.

Biegel, D.E. (1995) Caregiving, in *Encyclopedia of Disability and Rehabilitation*, Dell Orto, A.E. and Marinelli, R.P., Eds., Simon & Schuster/Macmillan, New York, 146–148.

Botuck, S. and Winsberg, B.G. (1991) Effects of respite on mothers of school-age and adult children with severe disabilities, *Ment. Retard.*, 29(1), 43–47.

Brown, B.W. and McCormick, T. (1988) Family coping following traumatic brain injury: an exploratory analysis with recommendations for treatment, *Fam. Relat.*, 37, 12–16.

Campbell, C.H. (1988) Needs of relatives and helpfulness of support groups in severe brain injury, *Rehabil. Nursing*, 13(6), 320–325.

Chwalisz, K. (1992) Perceived stress and caregiver burden after brain injury: a theoretical integration, *Rehabil. Psychol.*, 37(3), 189–203.

Chwalisz, K. (1996). The perceived stress model of caregiver burden: evidence from spouses of persons with brain injury, *Rehabil. Psychol.*, 41(2), 91–113.

Cohen, S. and Warren, R. (1985) *Respite Care*, Pro Ed, Austin, TX.

DeBoskey, D.S. (1996) *Coming Home: A Discharge Manual for Families of Persons with a Brain Injury*, HDI Publishers, Houston.

DeJong, G., Batavia, A.I., and Williams, J.M. (1990) Who is responsible for the lifelong well-being of a person with a brain injury?, *J. of Head Trauma*, 5(1), 9–22.

Dell Orto, A.E. (1988) Respite care: a vehicle for hope, the buffer against desperation, in *Family Interventions Throughout Chronic Illness and Disability*, Power, P.W., Dell Orto, A.E., and Gibbons, M., Eds., Springer, New York.

Dell Orto, A.E. and Power, P.W. (1994) *Head Injury and the Family: A Life and Living Perspective*, PMD Publishers, Winter Park, FL, 4, 5.

Durgin, C.J. (1989) Techniques for families to increase their involvement in the rehabilitation process, *Cognit. Rehabil.*, May/June, 22–25.

Gillen, R., Tennen, H., Affleck, G., and Steinpreis, R. (1998) Distress, depressive symtoms, and depressive disorder among caregivers of patients with brain injury, *J. of Head Trauma Rehabil.*, 13(3), 31–43.

Graff, S. and Minnes, P. (1989) Stress and coping in caregivers of persons with traumatic head injuries, *J. of Appl. Soc. Sci.*, 13(2), 293–316.

Grant, G. and McGrath, M. (1990) Need for respite-care services for caregivers of persons with mental retardation, *Am. J. of Ment. Retard.*, 94(6), 638–648.

Hegeman, K.M. (1987) A care plan for the family of a brain trauma client, *Rehabil. Nursing*, 13(5), 254–258.

Houts, P., Nezu. A., Nezu, C., and Bucher, J. (1996) The prepared family caregiver: A problem solving approach to family caregiving education, *Patient Ed. and Counseling*, 27, 63–73.

Jarman, D.J. and Stone, J.A. (1989) Brain injury: issues and benefits arising with a family support group, *Cognit. Rehabil.*, May/June, 30–32.

Kahana, E., Biegel, D.E., and Wykle, M.L., Eds. (1994) *Family Caregiving across the Life Span*, Newbury Park, CA.

Kane, R. and Penrod, J. (1995) *Family Caregiving in an Aging Society: Policy Perspectives*, Sage Publications, Thousand Oaks, CA.

Knop, D.S., Bergman-Evans, B., and Warton-McCabe, B. (1998) In sickness and in health: an exploration of the perceived quality of the marital relationship, coping, and depression in caregivers of spouses with Alzheimer's disease, *J. of Psychosoc. Nursing*, 36(1), 16–21.

Kosciulek, J. and Lustig, D. (1998) Predicting family adaptation from brain injury — related family stress, *J. of Appl. Rehabil. Counseling*, 29(1), 8–12.

Kreutzer, J., Gervasio, A., and Camplair, P. (1994) Patient correlates of caregiver's distress and family functioning after traumatic brain injury, *Brain Injury*, 8(3), 211–230.

Lawton, M.P., Brody, E.M., Saperstein, A., and Grimes, M. (1989) Respite services for caregivers: research findings for service planning, *Home Health Care Serv. Q.*, 10(1/2), 5–32.

Lefley, H. (1997) Synthesizing the family caregiving studies: implications for service planning, social policy, and further research, *Fam. Relat.*, 46, 443–450.

Levine, C. (1998) Rough crossings: family caregivers' odysseys through the health care system, United Hospital Fund, New York.

Levine, C. (1999) The loneliness of the long term caregiver, *The New England J. of Med.*, 340(20), 1587–1590.

Levine, C. and Zuckerman, C. (1999) The trouble with families: toward an ethic of accommodation, *Ann. of Intern. Med.*, 130, 148–152.

Lustig, D. (1999) Family caregiving of adults with mental retardation: key issues for rehabilitation, *J. of Rehabil.*, 65(2), 26–35.

Marks, R. (1987) The family dimension in long term care: an assessment of stress and intervention, *Pride Inst. J. of Long Term Home Health Care*, 6(2), 18–25.

McCubbin, H., Thompson, A., and McCubbin, M. (1996) Family assessment: resiliency, coping and adaptation — inventories for research and practice, University of Wisconsin, Madison, WI.

Mesibov, G.B. and Price, J.C. (1995) Respite care, in *Encyclopedia of Disability and Rehabilitation*, Dell Orto, A.E. and Marinelli, R.P., Eds., Simon & Schuster/Macmillan, New York.

Morris, R.G., Morris, L.W., and Britton, P.G. (1988) Factors affecting the emotional well being of the caregivers of dementia sufferers, *Br. J. of Psychiatr.*, 153, 147–156.

Oddy, M., Humphrey, M., and Uttley, D. (1978) Stresses upon the relatives of head-injured patients, *Br. J. of Psychiatr.*, 133, 507–513.

Pearson, M.A. and Deitrick, E.P. (1989) Support for family caregivers: a volunteer program for in-home respite care, *Caring*, 3(12), 18–20, 22.

Pullo, M.L. and Hahn, S. (1979) Respite care: a family support service, United Cerebral Palsy of Wisconsin, Inc., Madison, WI.

Ridley, B. (1989) Family response in brain injury: denial … or hope for the future?, *Soc. Sci. Med.*, 29(4), 555–561.

Rimmerman, A. (1989) Provision of respite care for children with developmental disabilities: changes in maternal coping and stress over time, *Ment. Retard.*, 27(2), 99–103.

Rosenthal, M. (1987) Traumatic brain injury: neurobehavioral consequences, in *Rehabilitation Psychology Desk Reference*, Caplan, B., Ed., Aspen, Rockville, MD, 37–63.

Rosenthal, M. and Young, T. (1988) Effective family intervention after traumatic brain injury: theory and practice, *J. of Head Trauma Rehabil.*, 3(4), 42–50.

Sander, A.M., High, W.M., Hanny, H.J., and Sherer, M. (1997) Relationship of coping style and social support to subjective burden and psychological health in caregivers of patients with closed head injury, *Brain Injury*, 11, 235–249.

Stroker, R. (1983). Impact of disability on families of stroke clients, *J. of Neurosurg. Nursing*, 15(6), 360–365.

Waaland, P.K. and Kreutzer, J.S. (1988). Family response to childhood traumatic brain injury, *J. of Head Trauma Rehabil.*, 3(4), 51–63.

Wallace, C.A., Bogner, J.A., Corrigan, J.D., Clinchot, D., Mysiw, W.J., and Fugate, L. (1998) Primary caregivers of persons with brain injury: life changes one year after injury, *Brain Injury*, 12, 483–493.

Wright, L.K. (1993) Alzheimer's Disease and Marriage: An Intimate Account, Sage Publications, Newbury Park, CA.

Zeigler, E.A. (1989) The importance of mutual support for spouses of brain injury survivors, *Cognit. Rehabil.*, May/June, 34–37.

chapter twelve

The future: hope, needs, and reality

Perspective

A primary theme of this book is that the family does not have to be destroyed by a brain injury — even if that is a reasonable outcome given the circumstances families must endure during onset, treatment, rehabilitation, and recovery.

Prior chapters have presented the impact of brain injury on the family from a living perspective which attempts to put the past in perspective and build a future enriched by optimism and opportunity. This final chapter will summarize some of the issues, address others, and introduce some myths related to brain injury. These are intended to be provocative and stimulate discussion and debate.

Brain injury transforms the entire family system. It has the power to confuse the present, distort the past, and challenge the future. It also creates familial stress and disappointment as well as healing and hope. Hope has emerged as an important consideration in the living process (Gottschalk, 1985; Nunn, 1996; Magaletta and Oliver, 1999; Scheier and Carver, 1992; 1998, Snyder et al., 1991) and is a vital force in the families' journeys to move beyond what was and begin to understand and accept what is and what could be.

Assisting families to cope with the emerging realities related to brain injuries is often a lifelong process. It demands the creative efforts of health and rehabilitation systems and their workers who are invested in and attuned to the needs of the person with a brain injury and the family. To expect the family to provide support implies that the health care and rehabilitation team are more than aware of the rigors of treatment, rehabilitation, and recovery. They must appreciate, comprehend, and value the costs and rewards of adjusting to a brain injury, as well as the importance of assisting the family to stabilize, recover, and grow. To facilitate the process of learning, coping, and surviving, the family needs timely and relevant interventions, appropriate skills, and accessible support. When these needs are met, the family's reactions to and decisions about the person with a brain injury, and themselves, can be made from a position of strength rather than desperation and frustration.

A harsh reality of life is that the occurrence of a brain injury is neither rational nor fair! However, this statement does not limit the reality of a brain injury experience in that it shatters dreams, destroys lives, changes families, and creates a complexity of health care issues which boggle the mind and rapidly deplete familial resources. Given the enormity and complexity of a brain injury, it would be easy to concede that the problems are too over-whelming for health care and family systems with limited resources, differ-ing priorities, and overwhelming needs.

This complexity is the driving force behind the brain injury movement which has set a course to meet the needs of families living brain injury experiences in spite of organizational obstacles, policy limitations, and com-peting interests. The challenge facing families, survivors, and health and human care providers is that it's not just a brain injury problem.

It is a human problem because all humans during their lives will expe-rience dynamic changes and major losses. Sometimes, there is a rational framework which facilitates the acceptance of this mortal reality, e.g., older persons who have reached retirement age, have lived fulfilling lives, dis-charged their responsibilities, and had their abilities altered by the normal conditions of aging.

The deterioration of an elderly person is a painful process, but it is more understandable than the randomness of most brain injuries which assault children, adolescents, and adults at the most inopportune times of their lives. This is compounded by the fact that most brain injuries are a result of choices, actions, and behaviors which make accepting the irreversible consequences of accidents, trauma, and irrational violence difficult at best and raises a multitude of complex issues (Banja and Johnston, 1994; Feldman, 1996; Cal-lahan, 1987; Phipps, 1998; Rosenthal and Lourie, 1996).

Currently the major focus is on the importance of outcomes related to brain injury rehabilitation (Hannay et al., 1996; Massagli et al., 1996; Cowen et al., 1995; Giacino and Zasler, 1995; Massagli et al., 1996; Hall, 1997; Watts and Perlesz, 1999; National Institute of Health, 1998; Perlesz, Kinsella, and Crowe, 1999; Rothweiler et al., 1998; Voogt et al.,1999; Zasler, 1997).

While there is value and importance in outcomes research, this informa-tion must be assessed and considered in the context of how it impacts families and their abilities to process, integrate, and benefit from the data and policy generated. This point is emphasized in a report from the Agency for Health Care Policy and Research (1998):

> Future research should focus on improving outcome measures used to examine the results of case manage-ment in TBI rehabilitation. In addition to outcomes of changed patient functionality, there should be out-comes of changed family functionality. Since much of case management communication is directed toward

> helping family members learn what to expect and where to obtain services, relevant outcomes would include family use of community and rehabilitation services and indicators of family assertiveness about care expectations. While case management may exert only an indirect effect on a patient's functional outcomes such as level of disability, vocational status, and living status, it is possible that case management can directly affect family knowledge of TBI rehabilitation needs and services, level of psychosocial anxiety, and family competency in coping with TBI (p. 8).

However, not everyone has the resources, support systems, or skills to negotiate a process that demands acceptance of an often overwhelming reality. Fortunately, there are people who are successfully surviving and managing life experiences which have been transformed and redefined by brain injuries.

For the family and person challenged by brain injury, this is an important realization because it demonstrates that in life, there are choices: people can choose to make the best out of a most difficult situation or not. In reality, though, is this always the case? It may sound good, but when discussing trauma, disability, or brain injury, it is essential to realize that families are often so emotionally and physically depleted they cannot make choices that are in their best interests. More often, decisions are made by default due to lack of support, role models, and skills needed to negotiate the demands and uncertainties of brain injury treatments and rehabilitation. In those situations where there are more familial problems than solutions, it is important to realize that some families are doing the very best they can with what they have have access to and the demands and expectations consequent to treatment and rehabilitation are far in excess of what they can do. For these families the issues are not non-compliance and disinterest but rather emotional hypothermia.

The challenge, therefore, is to approach brain injury treatment and rehabilitation from an optimistic and realistic perspective. This is not an easy task since there are many myths and forces which can influence expectations during the treatment and rehabilitation process. Rocchio (1998) has presented some myths related to family management of behavioral issues following brain injury. Some other general myths are:

Myth 1. Brain injury can be prevented

While it is a noble goal to reduce all of the precipitating and causal factors related to the incidence of brain injury, the reality is that no amount of education or prevention will eradicate all the variables that cause brain injury (e.g., drunk driving, drug-related violence, war, crime, accidents, sports injuries, abuse, work injuries, bicycles, etc.).

For those persons and families living with brain injuries, the past is unalterable, but the future can be somewhat controlled. The injury does exist and there is always the temptation to replay the reality while hoping for a different outcome. For those who bear witness to the tragedy of brain injuries, there is the drive and commitment to make sure that this does not occur to others or the family again, but as we all know, it will. In fact having a brain injury does not guarantee that a person will not have another. The possibility of another brain injury is actually increased, creating additional vigilance and concern for all involved. It is ironic that in some cases successful rehabilitation, increased independence, and expanded life domains may increase vulnerability to the very risks families are attempting to master and control. This is an ongoing complexity of life: there are no guarantees, only opportunities.

We cannot prevent the inevitable, but we must try to provide meaningful intervention, ongoing support, and caring. However, it is critical that all interventions be based on a realistic perspective of the human condition as it is and what it will become. People are in a constant state of growth and deterioration. We cannot be immunized from the human experience.

Brain injury is a tragedy for all who experience it. For some it is the greatest loss, for some it is bearable, and for others it is more positive than negative. Loss and change are undeniable dimensions and forces of the human experience. Consequently, every effort should be made to help the person and family live their lives with human dignity and values that appreciate life, accept mortality, recognize vulnerability, promote hope, and demonstrate caring. Some of the most poignant statements a family can make are, "we should have," "if only," "why us … ." Rarely do people say, "why not."

Myth 2. Restoration is more important than realistic acceptance

While significant gains have been made in brain injury prevention, treatment, and rehabilitation, there is still a void which cannot be filled but which must be accepted. This is the ultimate challenge for persons and families faced with the choice between retrieving who they were and accepting who they are now.

It is important that families are helped to recognize the difference between hope based on desperation and hope based on reality. For some families hope is what keeps them going and denial may be a means to keeping this hope alive. Rather than forcing the family to rush beyond where they are ready to be, there is a need to appreciate why they are where they are and facilitate the support that enables them to maximize their potential. This is where self-help organizations and groups can help develop functional perspectives for persons and families living in a twilight zone of confusion, pain, and overwhelming need. While the "storm" of brain injury may not be avoided, the accessibility to "safe harbors" can make surviving possible.

Myth 3. Someone must pay!

For many families enduring the journey of treatment and rehabilitation, this is an emotional and financial trap. Emotionally, a family may rightly feel they have been wronged — and often justifiably so. For example, a family may feel they've been wronged by a drunk driver whose actions placed a child in a coma management program. But what if this person is uninsured, a repeat offender, or has no resources? Who becomes the object of attention? Is it the media who promote alcohol use and abuse or the manufacturers who portray reckless driving in their ads? Is it the employer who unjustly fires a person who then becomes angry and shoots a co-worker which results in severe brain injury? What about the elderly driver whose poor skills and judgement caused a car accident and a subsequent brain injury of a child?

It is at this point when families are confused and angry for the wrong reason. The issue is not only who will pay, but what can be done to validate the injured person and make the life care process more reasonable. The problem is that no amount of money can regain what was lost, undo the pain and sorrow, and guarantee that life will be easier. While money can certainly relieve the financial burden and provide the resources needed to enhance quality of life, it can also cause additional problems.

Consider the reaction of a family awarded $2 million in a personal injury case for their brain-injured 17-year-old daughter. They bought her a sports car and as a result, she was in a car accident. She became a quadriplegic and her brother was killed. At this point, her mother stated that their situation went from bad to worse. The money promised a lot of hope, but delivered a great deal of pain. She added that they all would have been better off without it.

Large cash settlements have distorted the issues and created a caste system. Why should one person with a brain injury win a $5 million settlement and get the best of care while another lives in squalor with a broken wheelchair and without personal care attendants just because he was injured by a person without insurance, was indigent, or had diplomatic immunity? This is the real challenge of brain injury treatment, intervention, and policy. A system must be developed that is based upon human value, respect for life, and family stabilization. No cost is too great if it is helping those who have too little.

Myth 4. The family and person will always appreciate medical intervention

Another myth that creates stress for families is the expectation that all medical intervention is helpful and will be beneficial. When discussing brain injury, families and health care professionals must be able to discuss some very controversial, emotional, and unanswerable issues related to the cost, benefit, and effort related to intervention and outcome. For example, while some families are very happy that their family members' lives were saved even though there are severe limitations, other families may not be as pleased. This can change over time as the long-term reality of the situation is comprehended and the future is looming.

This point is well-illustrated by the anger and pain expressed by a mother who felt that the heroic efforts made by a medical team on a trauma helicopter did not save her son, but just prevented him from dying. Now both he and his family are relegated to an emotional and physical prison.

Apart from the financial costs and physical and emotional toll, the outcome has been individual stress and familial chaos. She is also very distressed with the legal and health care system that is profiting from the misery and suffering of her child, herself, and her family.

The emotionality and complexity of the issues related to cardiopulmonary resuscitation and the burden placed on families who are hoping for full recoveries while faced with losses are discussed by Phipps (1998).

> Because families view rehabilitation, at least initially, with a hopefulness for the patient's full recovery, initiating discussions of this topic early on in the rehabilitation process may be experiences as too emotionally burdensome to yield informed decisions and may be viewed as counterproductive to establishing trust and rapport. Some families appear to welcome talk about their own concerns, while others do not want to or are unable to grapple with the topic. Families who ultimately choose against resuscitation for their family member may have shifted in their hopefulness about the patient's recovery; may have lived with a patient with a chronic debilitating illness and believe that should the patient arrest, resuscitation may not be in the patient's best interest or possibly not in theirs" (p. 97).

An alternative perspective is the great appreciation families have for those heroic efforts which have kept their loved ones alive and have given them the chance to continue life but at a different level. As a wife stated in the personal statement in chapter five:

> One day I have a husband who is the strength of the family, who makes everyone proud and the next, I have this person who scares everyone with his temper and who thinks every thing is fine when it's a sorry mess.

> Life is getting better. The two of us get along. Sometimes I even like the fact that my husband is around all the time. He can be good company ... I guess we'll be a good old twosome until the day we die ... Life is hard. I'm a survivor.

In both of these examples, the common element is that the families are going to have to live with the consequences. The challenge for society and health care is to provide the support, encouragement, and role models needed to keep brain injury in perspective so that it does not become a ravaging force which destroys the family that is trying to survive.

Myth 5. Technology will provide all the answers

Without doubt, technology has enhanced the lives of people with brain injuries and has increased the options and opportunities in the life, learning, and working domains. However, for some families, what exists may not be relevant to the needs of their family members or may not be accessible. This creates a unique set of stressors for the person and family faced with conditions and situations that are not resolved by technology as it exists today.

Myth 6. Blind faith in the health care team and system

In some situations the needs of the family are secondary to the goals, interests, and resources of the people and systems involved in the care of a family member. This is often an alien concept for families who have looked toward these resources and systems from an overly optimistic frame of reference. Families must often advocate for themselves if they cannot align themselves with people and systems that can provide support.

Myth 7. Did not cause it, therefore not responsible

A lot of energy can be expended in focusing on the cause and circumstances related to the loss involved in a brain injury. When all is said and done the family may or may not be responsible for the cause but they have the opportunity to be responsible for the solution.

Conclusion

It is important to realize that a common goal most people share is to make the world a better place to live in within the constructs of a very individualized reality.

A major step in this process is recognizing that brain injury is another component in the continued exploration of our humanity. It is not the last challenge we will face as a society, but one of many emerging realities which will test our convictions, resources, and fortitude.

It is within a living perspective that many of the issues relative to brain injury treatment, rehabilitation, and recovery are cast into a different light. Brain injury will always be with us. So will hope, vision, and creativity. Approaching brain injury in a holistic, creative, and visionary way enhances the quality of life of the person living with brain injury and the family. The reality of brain injury can never be totally eliminated, but living with its consequences certainly can be made more bearable.

The following personal statement, *Making Dreams Come True, A Son's Perspective* captures the reality of living with a parent who was at one time considered immortal.

Personal statement

Making dreams come true, a son's perspective

All people have dreams, but few make the sacrifices to make those dreams come true. I read that on a poster once while waiting in a bus station to get home to see my father who was in a car accident. I wondered if I or my family had the ability to make the dream of my father's recovery a reality. To me, the situation was not believable or real.

My father seemed like an immortal man of 50, who not only loved life, but also challenged it. In his lifetime, he had been wounded in Vietnam and had recently recovered from a mild heart attack. The family believed that he could do anything he wanted to.

Our family was a high energy unit that enjoyed and celebrated life. While I was sitting in the bus station, I wondered if there would ever be cause for celebration again. When I arrived home, I found an overwhelming situation. My in-control family was completely out of control and looking to me as the eldest son for support and leadership. I was not prepared for this. All I wanted was to see my father and find him getting better. Unfortunately, he was near death and on life-support, and we were thrown into a state of shock and distress. At that point, I knew that me and my family had to focus our resources and help each other survive this most difficult situation. My mother expected and needed a miracle; she was certain he would recover. I was more pessimistic, while my brothers and sisters did not know what to do.

During the long months of hospitalization, we were told that the future was uncertain and that we should prepare ourselves to accept small gains if they occurred. Small gains did occur, then some bigger ones. In a sense, our father was emerging from the depths of the unknown and slowly he began to connect with the world around him. This was a small step in the right direction.

When dad returned home, in some ways he was his old self and in other ways he was a new person. His role as a family leader was taken over by my mother with the support of the family. The most helpful thing was that most people did not abandon us. My father's employer offered my younger brothers jobs and told my father he could have his job back when he got better. Even though this was unlikely, it gave us all a sense of hope.

For me and my family, the past 3 years have not been easy. Today, my father is living with the reality of his brain injury. At times, he is very difficult to live with. He is often inflexible, preoccupied with sports. This has been a major problem since the day he decided to stay home and watch the World

Series rather than go to his own daughter's wedding. While no one in the family could understand this decision, he still cannot comprehend why people were upset.

All in all, we are happy he is alive and wish the accident had not occurred. One thing we, as a family, agree is that it certainly could have been worse and it may even get better.

Discussion questions on the personal statement

1. How is the philosophy that "if you work hard at something, anything is possible" helpful or distressing for families coping with brain injuries?
2. What is meant by the statement "my father seemed an immortal man?"
3. In this case, could family expectations that their father could do anything create additional distress during rehabilitation?
4. What happens to a family that wants and needs a miracle and it does not happen?
5. Discuss the employer's response to this situation. Do you think this is typical or atypical?
6. What are the characteristics of this family which have enabled it to remain cohesive during the brain injury experience?

Set 17. Trauma helicopter

Perspective

Families are greatly relieved when family members survive the initial stages of trauma and are given the opportunity to continue life. This initial relief and joy often turns to distress and sadness when families realize that the people they knew left them when the brain injuries occurred, and now they are faced with the ongoing challenge of getting to know and accept people who are total or partial strangers. This often occurs when extraordinary and heroic efforts have less than normal results. While positive and miraculous outcomes result from most trauma rescue flights, some have created complex situations for families.

Exploration

1. Are there situations when medical care should be withheld at the scene of an accident?
2. How would you help a family enraged when a child was saved and must spend the rest of his or her life in a coma management unit?
3. Should a hospital or its personnel be responsible for the long-term care and financial costs if they resuscitate without the family's approval?

Set 18. Justice and injustice

Perspective

In the discussion on the concept of life care plans, there are three dimensions embodied in the terminology:

1. Life implies a biological component.
2. Care implies a beneficial interaction between recipients of care and caregivers.
3. Plan implies a carefully thought out sequence of decisions, acts, and consequences which have short and long-term positive benefits.

In discussing life care plans for persons and families living with brain injuries, there are other factors to be considered. Life may be empty or limited in quality, caring may be a myth driven by financial gain, and planning may be an overly detailed process which masks chaos and omits the flexibility needed to deal with changing systems.

Exploration

1. What are the essential elements of life care plans?
2. Should parents be required to return or be accountable for money awarded in settlements if they place the head-injured person in a public facility?
3. Should people who receive large settlements be required to contribute to the care of people who were brain-injured by uninsured drivers and left destitute?
4. How much money represents an adequate amount for the lifelong care of a brain-injured child?
5. Who should be responsible for the lifelong care of a severely brain-injured person if the family does not want to assume the role?
6. How much money is enough to compensate for a severe brain injury? How much money is too much?
7. Can brain injury be prevented?
8. Does the goal to make a person what he or she was before a brain injury interfere with the acceptance of who he or she is post injury?
9. What are the issues generated by the treatment and rehabilitation of a person with a brain injury who acquires AIDS as compared to a person with AIDS who acquires a brain injury?

References

Agency for Health Care Policy and Research (1998) Rehabilitation for Traumatic Brain Injury. Summary, Evidence Report/Technology Assessment, Portland, OR, Dec. 2.

Banja, J. and Johnston, M. (1994) Outcomes evaluation in TBI rehabilitation, part III, ethical perspectives in social policy, *Arch. of Phys. Med. and Rehabil.*, 75, 19–23.

Callahan, D. (1987) *Setting Limits: Medical Goals in an Aging Society,* Touchstone, New York.

Cowen, T., Meythaler, M., DeVivo, M., Ivie, C., Lebow, J., and Novack, T. (1995) Influence of early variables in traumatic brain injury on functional independence measure scores and rehabilitation length of stay and charges, *Arch. of Phys. Med. and Rehabil.*, 76, 800–803.

Dell Orto, A.E. and Power, P.W. (1994) *Head Injury and the Family: A Life and Living Perspective,* PMD Publishers, Winter Park, FL.

Feldman, Z. (1996) The limits of salvageability in head injury, in *Neuotrauma,* Narayan, R.K., Wilberger, J., and Povlishock, J., Eds., McGraw-Hill, New York, 805–817.

Giacino, J. and Zasler, N. (1995) Outcome after severe traumatic brain injury: coma the vegetative state and the minimally responsive state, *J. of Head Trauma Rehabil.*, 10, 40–56.

Gordon, W., Sliwinski, M., Echo, J., McLoughlin, M., Sheerer, M., and Meili, T.E. (1998) The benefits of exercise in individuals with traumatic brain injury: a retrospective study, *J. of Head Trauma Rehabil.*, 13(4), 58–67.

Gottschalk, L.A. (1985) Hope and other deterrents to illness, *Am. J. of Psychother.*, 39, 515–524.

Hall, K. (1997) Establishing a national traumatic brain injury information system based upon a unified data set, *Arch. of Phys. Med. and Rehabil.*, 78(8), S5–S11.

Hannay, H., Ezrachi, O., Contant, C., and Levin, H. (1996) Outcome measures for patients with head injuries: report of the outcome measures subcommittee, *J. of Head Trauma Rehabil.*, 11(6), 41–50.

Magaletta, P.R. and Oliver, J.M. (1999) The hope construct, wills and ways: their relations with self efficacy, optimism, and general well being, *J. of Clinical Psychol.*, 55(5), 539–551.

Massagli, T., Michaud, M., and Rivara, F. (1996) Association between injury indices and outcome after severe traumatic brain injury in children, *Arch. of Phys. Med. and Rehabil.*, 77, 125–131.

Nunn, K. (1996) Personal hopefulness: a conceptual review of the relevance of the perceive future to psychiatry, *Br. J. of Med. Psychol.*, 69, 227–245.

Perlesz, A., Kinsella, G., and Crowe, S. (1999) Impact of traumatic brain injury on the family: a critical review, *Rehabil. Psychol.*, 44(1), 6–35.

Phipps, E.J. (1998) Communication and ethics: cardiopulmonary resuscitation in head trauma rehabilitation, *J. of Head Trauma Rehabil.*, 13(5), 95–98.

National Institutes of Health (1998) Rehabilitation of persons with traumatic brain injury, Report of Consensus Development Conference, Oct., Bethesda, MD.

Rocchio, C. (1998) Can families manage behavioral programs in a home setting?, *Brain Injury Source*, 2(4), 34, 35.

Rosenthal, M. and Lourie, I. (1996) Ethical issues in the evaluation of competence in persons with brain injuries, *NeuroRehabil.*, 6(2), 113–121.

Rothweiler, B., Temkin, N., and Dikmen, S. (1998) Aging effect on psychosocial outcome in traumatic brain injury, *Arch. of Phys. Med. and Rehabil.*, 79(8), 881–887.

Scheier, M.F. and Carver, C.S. (1992) Effects of optimism or psychological and physical well being: theoretical overview and empirical update, *Cognit. Ther. and Res.*, 16, 201–228.

Scheier, M.F. and Carver, C.S. (1998) On the power of positive thinking: the benefits of being optimistic, *Curr. Directions in Psychol. Sci.,* 2, 26–30.

Snyder, C.R., Irving, L.M., and Anderson, J. (1991) Hope and health, in *Handbook of Social and Clinical Psychology,* Snyder, C.R. and Forsyth, D.R., Eds., Pergamon Press, Elmsford, NY, 285–305.

Voogt, R.D., Page,T., and Pennington, V. (1999) Real vs. clinical outcomes, *Brain Injury Source,* 3(2), 10–12.

Watts, R. and Perlesz, A. (1999) Psychosocial outcome risk indicator: predicting psychosocial outcome following traumatic brain injury, *Brain Injury,* 13(2), 113–124.

Zasler, N. (1997) Prognostic indicators in medical rehabilitation of traumatic brain injury: a commentary and review, *Arch. of Phys. Med. and Rehabil.,* 78, S12–S16.

Appendix A

Support groups and state associations of The Brain Injury Association*

Alabama
3600 8th Avenue South
Birmingham, AL 35222
(205) 328-3505
(800) 433-8002
Ahifl@aol.com

Alaska
1251 Muldoon Road, Suite 32
Anchorage, AK 99504
(907) 338-9800
(888) 945-HEAD
(907) 283-5711
www.alaska.net/~drussell/bia-ak/

Arizona
4545 N. 36th Street, Suite 125A
Phoenix, AZ 85018
(602) 952-2449
Fax: (602) 224-0010

Arkansas
PO Box 26236
Little Rock, AR 72221
(501) 771-5011
(800) 235-2443
Fax: (501) 227-8632

California
PO Box 160786
Sacramento, CA 95816-0786
(916) 442-1710
(800) 457-2443
Fax: (916) 442-7305
biac@juno.com

Colorado
6825 East Tennessee Avenue,
    Suite 405
Denver, CO 80224
(303) 355-9969
(800) 955-2443
Fax: (303) 355-9968
e-mail: biacolo@aol.com
www.BIAColorado.org

Connecticut
1800 Silas Deane Highway,
    Suite 224
Rocky Hill, CT 06067
(860) 721-8111
(800) 278-8242
Fax: (860) 721-9008
www.biact.org/

* With permission from The Brain Injury Association, Alexandria, VA.

213

Delaware
PO Box 479
Ocean View, DE 19970
(302) 537-5770
(800) 411-0505
Fax: 302-537-5770
www.biausa.org/Delaware/bia.
htm

Florida
North Broward Medical Center
201 East Sample Road
Pompano Beach, FL 33064
(954) 786-2400
(800) 992-3442
Fax: (954) 786-2437
BIAF@netrunner.net or
gatorbob@aol.com
www.biaf.org

Georgia
1447 Peachtree Street NE,
Suite 810
Atlanta, GA 30309
(404) 817-7577
(888) 334-2424
(404) 817-7521
BIAG@BrainInjuryGA.org
www.braininjuryga.org

Hawaii
1775 S. Beretania Street,
Suite 203
Honolulu, HI 96826
(808) 941-0372
biahi@cchono.com

Idaho
PO Box 414
Boise, ID 83701-0414
(208) 336-7708
(888) 374-3447
Fax: (208) 333-0026
melelina@aol.com

Illinois
1127 South Mannheim Road, Suite
213
Westchester, IL 60154
(708) 344-4646
(800) 699-6443
Fax: (708) 344-4680
biail@yahoo.com
www.biausa.org/Illinois/bia.htm

Indiana
15 North Ritter Avenue
Indianapolis, IN 46219
(317) 356-7722
(800) 407-4246
Fax: (317) 356-4241
biai@iquest.net
www.ohiovalley.org/HIFIhome.html

Iowa
2101 Kimball Avenue LL7
Waterloo, IA 50702
(319) 272-2312
(800) 475-4442
Fax: (319) 272-2109
edboll@mtcnet.net
www.biaia.org

Kansas
1100 Pennsylvania Ave., Suite 4061
Kansas City, MO 64105
(816) 842-8607
(800) 783-1356
(800) 783-3060
Fax: (816) 842-1531
elizabet@crn.org
www.brain-injury-ks-gkc.org

Kentucky
4229 Bardstown Rd., Suite 330
Louisville, KY 40207-3937
(502) 493-0609
(800) 592-1117
dir@braincenter.org
www.braincenter.org

Louisiana
217 Buffwood Drive
Baker, LA 70714-3755
(225) 775-2780
Fax: (225) 775-2780

Maine
211 Maine Ave., Suite 200
Farmingdale, ME 04344
(207) 582-4696
(800) 275-1233
Fax: (207) 582-4803
Biaofme@ctrl.net
www.biausa.org/Maine/bia.
  htm

Maryland
Kernan Hospital
2200 Kernan Drive
Baltimore, MD 21207
(410) 448-2924
(800) 221-6443
Fax: (410) 448-3541
biamaryland@erols.com
www.biamd.org

Massachusetts
Denholm Building
484 Main Street, Suite 325
Worcester, MA 01608
(508) 795-0244
(800) 242-0030
Fax: (508) 757-9109
Mbia1@ma.ultranet.com
www.mbia.net

Michigan
8619 W. Grand River, Suite I
Brighton, MI 48116-2334
(810) 229-5880
(800) 772-4323
Fax: (810) 229-8947
BIAOFMI@cac.net
www.concentic.net/~biami

Minnesota
43 Main Street SE, Suite 135
Minneapolis, MN 55414
(612) 378-2742
(800) 669-6442
Fax: (612) 378-2789
biam@protocom.com
www.braininjurymn.org

Mississippi
PO Box 55912
Jackson, MS 39296-5912
(601) 981-1021
(800) 641-6442
Fax: (601) 981-1039
biaofms@aol.com
www.members.aol.com/biaofms/
  index.htm

Missouri
10270 Page, Suite 100
St. Louis, MO 63132
(314) 426-4024
(800) 377-6442
Fax: (314) 426-3290
braininjry@aol.com
www.biausa.org/bia.htm

Montana
52 Corbin Hall RM. 333
Missoula, MT 59812
(406) 243-5973
(800) 241-6442
Fax: (406) 243-2349
biam@selway.umt.edu

Nebraska
PO Box 124
Gothenburg, NE 69138
(308) 537-7875/537-7663
(888) 642-4137
Fax: (308) 537-7663
bi13135@navix.net
www.biausa.org/Nebraska/bia.htm

Nevada (Northern)
PO Box 2789
Gardnervill, NV 89410
(702) 782-8336

Nevada (Southern)
2820 W. Charleston Boulevard,
    Suite D-37
Las Vegas, NV 89102
(702) 259-1903

New Hampshire
2 1/2 Beacon Street
Concord, NH 03301-4447
(603) 225-8400
(800) 773-8400
Fax: (603) 228-6749
nhbia@nh.ultranet.com
www.bianh.org

New Jersey
1090 King George Post Road,
    Suite 708
Edison, NJ 08837
(732) 738-1002
(800) 669-4323
Fax: (732) 738-1132
info@bianj.org
www.bianj.org

New Mexico
11000 Candelaria NE, Suite 113-W
Albuquerque, NM 87112
(505) 292-7414
(888) 292-7415
Headwaynm@aol.com

New York
10 Colvin Avenue
Albany, NY 12206-1242
(518) 459-7911
(800) 228-8201
Fax: (518) 482-5285
info@bianys.org   or
    javner@bianys.org
www.bianys.org

North Carolina
PO Box 748
Raleigh, NC 27602
(919) 833-9634
(800) 377-1464
Fax: (919) 833-5415
biaofnc@aol.com or
    cbgreene@aol.com
www.bianc.org

North Dakota
Open Door Center
Valley City, ND 58072
(701) 845-1124
Fax: (701) 845-1175

Ohio
1335 Dublin Road,
    Suite 217D
Columbus, OH 43215-1000
(614) 481-7100
(800) 686-9563
Fax: (614) 481-7103
help@biaoh.org
www.biaoh.org

Oklahoma
PO Box 88
Hillsdale, OK 73743-0088
(580) 635-2237
(800) 765-6809
Fax: (580) 635-2238
biaok@ionet.net
www.ionet.net/~rxot/

Oregon
1118 Lancaster Drive,
    NE – PMB 301
Salem, OR 97301-2933
(503) 585-0855
(800) 544-5243
Fax: (503) 589-1869
biaor@open.org
www.open.org/~biaor/

Pennsylvania (East)
(800) 383-8889
www.libertynet.org/bia-e-pa

Pennsylvania (West)
304 Morewood Avenue
Pittsburgh, PA 15213
(412) 682-2520
Charlotteherbert@msn.com
www.biausa.org/wPenn/
    index.htm

Rhode Island
Independence Square —
    500 Prospect
Pawtucket, RI 02860
(401) 725-2360
Fax: (401) 727-2810
BuckleUp1@aol.com
www.oso.com/community/
    groups/brain/index.html

South Carolina
(currently known as the South
    Carolina Brain Injury Task
    Force)
1030 St. Andrews Road
Columbia, SC 29210
(803) 731-0588
(800) 290-6461
Fax: (803) 731-0589
Scbraininjury@mindspring.
    com

Tennessee
699 W. Maine Street, Suite
    203B
Hendersonville, TN 37075
(423) 974-6713
(800) 480-6693
Fax: (615) 264-1693
BIAofTN@hotmail.com
home.earthinlink.net/~BIAT

Texas
1339 Lamar Square Drive,
    Suite C
Austin, TX 78704
(512) 326-1212
(800) 392-0040
Fax: (512) 326-8088
info@biatx.org

Utah
1800 S West Temple, Suite 203,
    Box 22
Salt Lake City, UT 84115
(801) 484-2240
(800) 281-8442
Fax: (801) 484-5932
biau@sisna.com
www.starpage.com/braininjury

Vermont
128 Prim Road, Suite 3A
Colchester, VT 05466
(802) 658-5600
Fax: (802) 658-5805
Vtbia@aol.com

Virginia
3212 Cutshaw Avenue, Suite 315
Richmond, VA 23230
(804) 355-5748
(800) 334-8443
Fax: (804) 355-6381
biav@visi.net
www.bia.pmr.vcu.edu/

Washington
16315 NE 87th, Suite B-4
Redmond, WA 98052-3537
(425) 895-0047
(800) 523-5438
Fax: (425) 895-0458
biawa@biawa.org
www.biawa.org

Washington D.C.
2100 Mayflower Drive
Lake Ridge, VA 22192
(202) 877-1464
Fax: (202) 291-5366

West Virginia
PO Box 574
Institute, WV 25112-0574
(304) 766-4892
(800) 356-6443
Fax: (304) 766-4940
biawv@aol.com
www.biaus.org/wvirginia

Wisconsin
3505 N. 124th St., Suite 100
Brookfield, WI 53005
(414) 790-6901
(800) 882-9282
Fax: (414) 790-6824

Wyoming
246 South Center, Suite 16
Casper, WY 82601
(307) 473-1767
(800) 643-6457
Fax: (307) 237-5222
biaw@trib.com

Appendix B

Selected resources

TBI Model Systems

National Institute on Disability and Rehabilitation Research
Washington, D.C.
www.ed.gov/office/OSERS/NIDRR/

The Traumatic Brain Injury Model Systems National Data Center
Kessler Medical Rehabilitation Research and Education Corporation
West Orange, New Jersey
www.kmrrec.org

University of Alabama at Birmingham
Spain Rehabilitation Center
Birmingham, Alabama
www.uab.edu/tbi

Santa Clara Valley Medical Center
San Jose, California
www.tbi-sci.org or www.tbi-sci.org/rehab

Craig Hospital
Englewood, Colorado
www.craighospital.org

Emory University
Shepherd Center
Atlanta, Georgia
www.emory.edu

The Spaulding Rehabilitation Hospital
Boston, Massachusetts
www.spauldingrehab.org

Southeastern Michigan Traumatic Brain Injury System
Wayne State University/Rehabilitation Institute of Michigan
Detroit, Michigan
www.semtbis.org

Mayo Foundation
Rochester, Minnesota
www.mayo.edu/model-system

TBI Model System of Mississippi
Mississippi Methodist Hospital and Rehabilitation Center
Jackson, Mississippi
www.mmrcrehab.org

University of Missouri
Columbia, Missouri
www.hsc.missouri.edu/~mombis

Kessler Medical Rehabilitation Research and Education Corporation
West Orange, New Jersey
www.kmrrec.org

Charlotte Institute of Rehabilitation
Chrlotte-Mecklenburg Hospital Authority
Charlotte, North Carolina
www.charweb.org/health/rehab/

The Ohio State University
Columbus, Ohio
www.ohiovalley.org/

Oregon Health Sciences University
Portland, Oregon
www.ohsu.edu

Moss Rehabilitation Research Institute
Philadelphia, Pennsylvania
www.einstein.edu/phl/1217p.html

The Institute for Rehabilitation and Research
Houston, Texas
www.tmc.edu/tirr/tirr-tirr_facts.html

Medical College of Virginia
Richmond, Virginia
www.neuro.pmr.vcu.edu/

University of Washington
Seattle, Washington
www.depts.washington.edu/rehab/

Other Internet Links

TBI-Net (Mount Sinai Rehabilitation Medicine)
Research and Training Center (RTC) on Community Integration of Individuals with Traumatic Brain Injury.
www.mssm.edu/tbinet/

The National Rehabilitation Information Center (NARIC)
Browse NARIC Database on Brain Injuries.
www.naric.com

Brain Injury Association, Inc. (BIA)
The mission of the Brain Injury Association is to promote awareness, understanding and prevention of brain injury through eduction, advocacy, research grants and community support services that lead toward reduced incidence and improved outcomes of children and adults with brain injuries.
www.biausa.org

RRTC on Rehabilitation Interventions in Traumatic Brain Injury
The Institute for Rehabilitation and Research (TIRR)
www.tirr.org/research/brain.html

Appendix C

Selected books

Acquired Brain Injury in Childhood and Adolescence: A Team and Family Guide to Education Program Development and Implementation
Alan L. Goldberg, Ed., C. Thomas, 1997

Brain Injury: A Family Tragedy
Patt Abrahamson and Jeffery Abrahamson, HDI, 1997

Brain Injury Rehabilitation: The Role of the Family in TBI Rehab (HDI Professional Series, Vol. 19)
Mark L. Guth, et al., HDI 1996

Children With Acquired Brain Injury: Educating and Supporting Families (Families, Community and Disability, Vol. 2)
George H. S. Singer, Ann Glang, and Janet Williams, Eds., 1996

Coming Home: A Discharge Manual for Families of Persons with a Brain Injury
D. S. DeBoskey, HDI, 1996

Coping With Brain Injury: A Guide for Family and Friends
Gordon Giles, Ed., American Occupational Therapy Association, 1996

Coping with Mild Traumatic Brain Injury
D. R. Stoler and B. A. Hill, Avery, 1998

Families, Illness and Disability
J. S. Rolland, BasicBooks, 1994

Family Support Programs and Rehabilitation: A Cognitive-Behavioral Approach to Traumatic Brain Injury (Critical Issues in Neuropsychology)
Louise Margaret Smith, Hamish P.D. Godfrey, Plenum Press, 1995

Head Injury: A Family Matter
J. M. Williams and T. Kay, Eds., Paul H. Brooks, 1991

Independent Living and Brain Injury
  J. M. Williams and M. Mathews, Research and Training Center on Independent Living for Undeserved Populations, University of Kansas, 1998

Living with Brain Injury: A Guide for Families and Caregivers
  Sonia Griffin Acorn and Penny Offer, University of Toronto Press, 1998

Management of Brain Injured Children
  R. Appleton and T. Baldwin, Oxford University Press, 1998

Psychotherapeutic Interventions for Adults with Brain Injury or Stroke: A Clinician's Treatment Resource
  Karen Langer, Linda Laatsch, and Lisa Lewis, Psychosocial Press, 1999

Rehabilitation of the Adult and Child with Traumatic Brain Injury
  M. Rosenthal, E. Griffith, J. Kreutzer, and B. Pentland, 3rd ed., F.A. Davis, 1998

Sexuality and Acquired Brain Injury in Children and Adolescents: A Guide for Health Professionals and the Family
  Helen Dawson et al., New Children's Hospital, Sydney, Australia, 1999

Treating Families of Brain-Injured Survivors (Springer Series on Rehabilitation, Vol., 9)
  Paul R. Sachs, 1991

Index

A

G

H